PROGRESS IN CLINICAL AND BIOLOGICAL RESEARCH

RECENT TITLES

Please contact the publisher for information about previous titles in this series.

PREDICTION OF RESPONSE TO CANCER THERAPY

PREDICTION OF RESPONSE TO CANCER THERAPY

Proceedings of a Symposium Held at the XVth International Chemotherapy
Congress, Istanbul, Turkey, July 19–24, 1987

Editor

Thomas C. Hall
Center for Molecular Medicine
and Immunology
University of Medicine and
Dentistry of New Jersey
Newark, New Jersey

ALAN R. LISS, INC. • NEW YORK

Library of Congress Cataloging-in-Publication Data

Prediction of response to cancer therapy.

 (Progress in clinical and biological research ;
v. 276)
  1. Cancer—Chemotherapy—Evaluation—Congresses.
2. Cancer—Prognosis—Congresses.   I. Hall, Thomas C.,
1921–   .   II. International Congress of Chemotherapy
(15th : 1987 : Istanbul, Turkey)   III. Series.
[DNLM: 1. Neoplasms—therapy—congresses.   2. Prognosis—
congresses.   WI PR668E v.276 / QZ 266 P9234 1987]
RC271.C5P729 1988   616.99′406   88-9392
ISBN 0-8451-5126-6

Contents

Contributors

Matti S. Aapro, Division d'Onco-Hématologie, Hôpital Cantonal Universitaire, 1211 Geneva 4, Switzerland **[255]**

Betty J. Abbott, Developmental Therapeutics Program, Division of Cancer Treatment, National Cancer Institute, Bethesda, MD 20892 **[265]**

Osahiko Abe, Department of Surgery, School of Medicine, Keio University, Shinjuku-ku, Tokyo 160, Japan **[213]**

Jaffer A. Ajani, Department of Medical Oncology, Division of Medicine, University of Texas M.D. Anderson Hospital and Tumor Institute, Houston, TX 77030 **[105]**

Joseph C. Allegra, Department of Medicine, James Graham Brown Cancer Center, University of Louisville, Louisville, KY 40292 **[11]**

Michael C. Alley, Developmental Therapeutics Program, Division of Cancer Treatment, National Cancer Institute, Bethesda, MD 20892 **[265]**

Fraser L. Baker, Department of Experimental Radiotherapy, Division of Radiotherapy, University of Texas M.D. Anderson Hospital and Tumor Institute, Houston, TX 77030 **[105]**

Arthur E. Bogden, Biomeasure Incorporated/Bogden Laboratories, Hopkinton, MA 01748 **[139]**

Michael R. Boyd, Developmental Therapeutics Program, Division of Cancer Treatment, National Cancer Institute, Bethesda, MD 20892 **[265]**

William A. Brock, Department of Experimental Radiotherapy, Division of Radiotherapy, University of Texas M.D. Anderson Hospital and Tumor Institute, Houston, TX 77030 **[105]**

William R. Cobb, Biomeasure Incorporated/Bogden Laboratories, Hopkinton, MA 01748 **[139]**

Maria Grazia Daidone, Oncologia Sperimentale C, Istituto Nazionale per lo Studio e la Cura dei Tumori, 20133 Milan, Italy **[93]**

Thomas G. Day, Jr., Department of Obstetrics and Gynecology, James Graham Brown Cancer Center, University of Louisville, Louisville, KY 40292 **[11]**

William L. Dean, Department of Biochemistry, James Graham Brown Cancer Center, University of Louisville, Louisville, KY 40292 **[11]**

The numbers in brackets are the opening page numbers of the contributors' articles.

Thomas E. Duarte, Veterans Administration Medical Center, Long Beach, CA **[75]**

J.F. Eliason, Department of Cellular Biology, I.S.R.E.C., 1066 Epalinges, Switzerland **[255]**

Donald L. Fine, Program Resources Inc., National Cancer Institute-Frederick Cancer Research Facility, Frederick, MD 21701 **[265]**

Emil J Freireich, Adult Leukemia Research Program, The University of Texas System Cancer Center, M.D. Anderson Hospital and Tumor Institute, Houston, TX 77030 **[227]**

Suzanne A.W. Fuqua, Department of Medicine/Oncology, University of Texas Health Science Center at San Antonio, San Antonio, TX 78284-7884 **[61]**

Uri Galili, MacMillan-Cargill Hematology Research Laboratory, Cancer Research Institute, The University of California, San Francisco, CA 94143 **[43]**

Matti Grönroos, Clinic of Obstetrics and Gynecology, Turku, Finland **[205]**

Thomas C. Hall, The Center for Molecular Medicine and Immunology, Newark, NJ 07103 **[xiii,1,295]**

Thomas C. Hamilton, Experimental Therapeutics Section, Medicine Branch, National Cancer Institute, Bethesda, MD 20892 **[287]**

Pähr-Einar Hellström, Meltola Hospital, Turku, Finland **[205]**

C. Herman, Department of Pathology, Loyola University, Maywood, IL 60153 **[255]**

Steven M. Hill, Department of Medicine/Oncology, University of Texas Health Science Center at San Antonio, San Antonio, TX 78284-7884 **[61]**

Kyuya Ishibiki, Department of Surgery, School of Medicine, Keio University, Shinjuku-ku, Tokyo 160, Japan **[213]**

Lauri Kangas, Farmos Group, Research Center, 20101 Turku, Finland **[205]**

Hannu Käpylä, Farmos Group, Research Center, 20101 Turku, Finland **[205]**

Tetsuro Kubota, Department of Surgery, School of Medicine, Keio University, Shinjuku-ku, Tokyo 160, Japan **[213]**

Doreen J. LePage, Biomeasure Incorporated/Bogden Laboratories, Hopkinton, MA 01748 **[139]**

Juhani Mäenpää, Clinic of Obstetrics and Gynecology, Turku, Finland **[205]**

Joseph G. Mayo, Developmental Therapeutics Program, Division of Cancer Treatment, National Cancer Institute, Bethesda, MD 20892 **[265]**

William L. McGuire, Department of Medicine/Oncology, University of Texas Health Science Center at San Antonio, San Antonio, TX 78284-7884 **[61]**

Theodore L. McLemore, Developmental Therapeutics Program, Division of Cancer Treatment, National Cancer Institute, Bethesda, MD 20892 **[265]**

Douglas E. Merkel, Department of Medicine/Oncology, University of Texas Health Science Center at San Antonio, San Antonio, TX 78284-7884 **[61]**

Anne Monks, Program Resources Inc., National Cancer Institute-Frederick Cancer Research Facility, Frederick, MD 21701 **[265]**

Robert A. Nagourney, University of California at Irvine, Irvine, CA and Oncotech, Inc., Irvine, CA 92714 **[75]**

Robert F. Ozols, Experimental Therapeutics Section, Medicine Branch, National Cancer Institute, Bethesda, MD 20892 **[287]**

Kenneth D. Paull, Developmental Therapeutics Program, Division of Cancer Treatment, National Cancer Institute, Bethesda, MD 20892 **[265]**

Renate Pelka-Fleischer, Medical Clinic III, Ludwig-Maximilians-Universität, Munich and Institute of Clinical Hematology GSF, Munich, Federal Republic of Germany **[237]**

Seppo Pyrhönen, Radiotherapy Clinic, Finland **[205]**

Peter Roberts, Turku University Central Hospital, IV Surgical Clinic, Turku, Finland **[205]**

Timo Romppanen, Kontioniemi Hospital, Finland **[205]**

Marcel Rozencweig, Clinical Cancer Research, Bristol Myers, Wallingford, CT 06492-7660 **[255]**

Youcef M. Rustum, Department of Experimental Therapeutics, Grace Cancer Drug Center, Roswell Park Memorial Institute, Buffalo, NY 14263 **[119]**

Pekka Saarelainen, Meltola Hospital, Turku, Finland **[205]**

Ornella Sanfilippo, Oncologia Sperimentale C, Istituto Nazionale per lo Studio e la Cura dei Tumori, 20133 Milan, Italy **[93]**

Hansjörg Sauer, Medical Clinic III, Ludwig-Maximilians-Universität, Munich and Institute of Clinical Hematology GSF, Munich, Federal Republic of Germany **[237]**

Dominic A. Scudiero, Program Resources Inc., National Cancer Institute-Frederick Cancer Research Facility, Frederick, MD 21701 **[265]**

Robert H. Shoemaker, Developmental Therapeutics Program, Division of Cancer Treatment, National Cancer Institute, Bethesda, MD 20892 **[265]**

Rosella Silvestrini, Oncologia Sperimentale C, Istituto Nazionale per lo Studio e la Cura dei Tumori, 20133 Milan, Italy **[93]**

Harry K. Slocum, Department of Experimental Therapeutics, Grace Cancer Drug Center, Roswell Park Memorial Institute, Buffalo, NY 14263 **[119]**

Gary Spitzer, Department of Hematology, Division of Medicine, University of Texas M.D. Anderson Hospital and Tumor Institute, Houston, TX 77030 **[105]**

Yong-zhuang Su, University of California at Irvine, Irvine, CA **[75]**

Lauri Tammilehto, Department of Pulmonary Medicine, Helsinki University Central Hospital, Helsinki, Finland **[205]**

Liane Twardzik, Medical Clinical III, Ludwig-Maximilians-Universität, Munich and Institute of Clinical Hematology GSF, Munich, Federal Republic of Germany **[237]**

M. Uitendaal, Department of Pharmacology, University of Limburg, 6200 MD Maastricht, The Netherlands **[255]**

Alexander van Assendelft, Kontioniemi Hospital, Finland **[205]**

Ursula Vehling-Kaiser, Medical Clinic III, Ludwig-Maximilians-Universität, Munich and Institute of Clinical Hematology GSF, Munich, Federal Republic of Germany **[237]**

Larry M. Weisenthal, Veterans
Administration Medical Center, Long
Beach, CA and University of California
at Irvine, Irvine, CA; present address:
Oncotech Inc., Irvine, CA 92714 **[75]**

Wolfgang Wilmanns, Medical Clinic
III, Ludwig-Maximilians-Universität,
Munich and Institute of Clinical
Hematology GSF, Munich, Federal
Republic of Germany **[237]**

James L. Wittliff, Department of
Biochemistry, James Graham Brown
Cancer Center, University of Louisville,
Louisville, KY 40292 **[11]**

Robert C. Young, Experimental
Therapeutics Section, Medicine Branch,
National Cancer Institute, Bethesda,
MD 20892 **[287]**

Nadia Zaffaroni, Oncologia
Sperimentale C, Istituto Nazionale per
lo Studio e la Cura dei Tumori, 20133
Milan, Italy **[93]**

Preface

This volume represents the proceedings of a symposium that was part of the International Chemotherapy Congress held in Istanbul in July 1987. This was the second such international meeting dealing with the broad spectrum of cancer therapies, the first having been held in Williamsburg, Virginia, in 1970. During the past 18 years, our understanding has progressed concerning the greater complexity of response prediction for tumors than for infectious agents. We have seen the coming and going of dye exclusion and soft-agar tests and the increasing realization that a panel of models is probably necessary for full prognostic evaluation.

Thomas C. Hall

Prediction of Response to Cancer Therapy, pages 1-9
© 1988 Alan R. Liss, Inc.

PURPOSES, BENEFITS AND TECHNIQUES OF CANCER TREATMENT
PREDICTIVE TESTS

Thomas C. Hall, M.D.

The Center for Molecular Medicine and
Immunology, Newark, NJ

Introduction

The clinical oncologist has a number of therapeutic
agents available which are about the same in number as
those used by the infectious disease specialist. However,
the frequency of responses by cancers to any drug or combination is far less than for the infected patient, and the
clinical relapse rate and emergence of drug resistance is
much higher for cancers. Thus, the need for tests predictive of responses is numerically greater in Oncology, but
the number of effective tests is lower. The ability to
avoid using ineffective cancer drugs and to create combinations including the most effective ones is desirable, fig
(1). Thus, the prime goal of a predictive test is improved
individualization of therapy for a patient by the clinician. A second major goal is to identify new drugs with
some overall antitumor effect from amongst the many
candidates that are continually being developed. This goal
is of interest to institutional drug developers such as the
National Cancer Institute, pharmaceutical companies, cancer
centers, and schools of pharmacy and medicine. In addition
to the obvious benefits, the design of an effective drug
screening predictive system would also decrease expense,
and useless toxicity, increase goodness of fit between drug
and tumor type, encourage new drug development, decrease
time to clinical trials and save lives.

Screens that individualize patient care have been
called "patient-oriented" or "clinical". Those that

Figure 1
Benefits from Predictive Tests

+Response Prediction

1. Increased quantity of life
2. Increased quality of life
3. Avoid unnecessary toxicity
4. Which 2nd line Rx to Choose

(-) Failure Prediction

1. Omit ineffective but toxic drugs
2. Decrease number of drugs in combinations
3. Avoid delay due to ineffective drugs
4. Decreased expense - dollars
                      - psychic
5. Speed new drug trials

assist in identification of effective new drugs have been
called "drug oriented" or "pharmacologic". However in the
past, the mouse tumors against which new drugs are tried
were chosen because they were easily transplantable, sensitive to clinical doses of drugs, and had been shown to predict in a general way for later clinical response. Most of
the screens were intraperitoneal mouse leukemias, and had
the often felicitous, if not entirely explicable, feature
of choosing drugs that later were found to be effective for
solid human tumor treated by the oral or intravenous
routes. However, only 100 or so agents were found out of
several hundred thousand tested, and there is always the
concern that some compounds which were inactive in mouse
tumors, might have been good for human patients.

Many predictive tests that have been developed can
also be thought of as "constitutive" i.e. they measure a
capacity or quality or feature of the tumor which predicts
that this tumor in this patient will respond to this or
these specific therapies. Such analyses are done on the
tumor tissue itself, and do not involve transplantation of
the tumor to a new place in which to grow, or observation
of the tumor-drug interaction over time. Examples include
those for the presence of drug receptors, the rate of
inward or outward drug transport, the amount of GSH or
phosphorylating enzymes. The other type of test is
"perturbational": the effects of drug treatment on the

target tumor are examined over a short time (hours to weeks), in the host, or more commonly in vitro or in special animal system. All the new drug preclinical selection screens have been "perturbational", and most human predictive tests have related to drugs in ways that are both constitutive and perturbational.

The usual pharmacologic triad; of drug, tumor and host operates also in the predictive testing situation, since these are only anticipatory microcosms of clinical treatment. However, the predictive system itself adds distortions from or modifications of the usual triad. In the next paragraphs we shall look at these variables in some detail, and the overall format of this volume will also reflect these factors.

A. Drug types make differing demands upon screening systems: 1) antimetabolities such as methotrexate require the tumor to be able to transport them across the plasma membrane. In addition, they are mitotoxic and act best upon rapidly replicating DNA in tumors with high growth fractions. Thus, the end point of the test can be a change in the net synthesis of new DNA over a few hours, or the lack of increase in numbers of cells, "growth" or "clonogenicity", over days to weeks. 2) Alkylating agents, while they are mitotoxic, also may have immediate beneficial effects against slowly dividing tumor cells such as the chronic leukemias, lymphomas, and sarcomas. In these circumstances, "cytotoxics" that kill non-dividing cells by intoxicating overall metabolism may be analyzed over a few hours following drug exposure and the end points may be "non clonogenic", e.g., decreased glycolysis, altered membrane permeability or cell lysis. 3) The plant natural products and the antibiotics commonly act against both the dividing cells, e.g. leukemia, and slowly dividing e.g. sarcoma cells. Thus a broadly applicable predictive test may need to deal with a spectrum of drugs with both modes of action. 3) For steroids, tests for clonogenicity or cell number change can measure both cytoxic and mitotoxic drug effects. But steroids also may lyse cells, as in the case of corticoids, or promote terminal differen-tiation, (high dose estrogen and progestins), or interfere with tumor proliferation caused by the endogenous steroids of the host (antiestrogens). Measuring each of these functions in vitro would be a difficult task, but fortu-nately a constitutive element of the tumor cell--the

cycloplasmic steroid receptor can be assayed as a predictor
for all of the steroid actions. 4) Cisplatin activity can
be related to the level of glutathione, and probably other
reducing agents, constitutive in the target tumors. 5)
Asparaginase seems to be effective when there is a tumor
requirement for an adequate ambient concentration of the
amino acid. However, this drug may cause toxicity to
normal tissues by the same mechanism and; hence, it may be
necessary for a useful system to predict host toxicity,
this may require sampling both normal tissues and tumors.
As a general rule, preclinical screening systems have been
weakened by the absence of determinations of effects on
normal tissues.

In many clinical situations, knowledge of the route of
administration may be of help, since this bears upon the
drug concentrations to be tested: intrathecal methotrexate causes substantial CNS side effects, and these
might be minimized if the lowest cytotoxic concentration to
tumor cells could be predicted and chosen. A very important consideration for predictive test development lies in
the current use of combination therapy. Multiple, simultaneous and sequential therapy has greatly increased the numbers and duration of clinical responses. However, every
drug added to a combination carries a high likelihood of
increased toxicity, with a much smaller likelihood of benefit. Single drugs that could be predicted as ineffective
for a patient could be dropped from combinations or replaced with others predicted to have benefit. Predictive
tests that would indicate the duration of cytotoxicity
following drug exposures would permit rational combinations
to be built and implemented at the optimal time intervals.
So far, in vitro tests have been relatively unable to provide information about drug combinations, dose levels or
sequences. The subcapular renal assay is limited to a
six-day period, but works well for combinations. Probably
the best assay to select the optimal frequency of dosing is
the nude mouse xenografted with fresh human tumor tissue
obtained at operation.

B. Type of tumor is very important. Hematologic
malignancies and respiratory solid tumors have not grown
well enough in the clonogenic agar tests for them to be
applicable. The fixed-phase cultures reportedly work
better and may permit the addition of growth factors that
will increase the yield of cells and their response to

treatment. For some hematologic malignancies, drug responsiveness can be predicted by initial histological, karyotypic, and histochemical characterizations. Recently the presence of specific cytologic changes such as chromosomal deletions of q5 and q7 have been associated with valid predictions for drug resistance. In some instances, a high level of oncogene product in tumor biopsies has been used to predict poor drug sensitivity. The use of cell separation has resulted in understanding of both overall replication rate and the predictive value of abnormalities in ploidy. For any assay, the use of isolates from cells growing in malignant effusions results in higher yields and better predictions. Simple factors such as size of the biopsy specimen, degrees of necrosis, and heterogeneity, both from infiltrating stromal cells and varying degrees of forward differentiation toward normality, all infringe on the validity of the tests.

C. Host factors such as previous therapy are known to effect the drug responsiveness of residual or recurrent tumor, and thus also the drugs selected for use in the test system. The need for a good prediction system to select second line drugs may be greater than for selection of initial therapy, since much initial therapy is dictated by what is proven and practical. For many tumors, such as leukemia and lymphoma, breast, ovary, small cell lung cancer, the response to conventional initial combinations is so high as to cast doubt on the need for an initially predictive test. However, a predictive test for the selection of drugs in relapsed patients is badly needed.

The host provides many hints as to what treatments could be effective, and when a poor prognosis for conventional therapy justifies aggressive or experimental therapy. Dr. Freireich discusses these clinical predictive "global" features extensively. Age of host affects both tumor types diagnosed, which in turn affects the viability of tissues in test systems. Age of host also relates to relative drug resistance of the host tissues to drug therapy, i.e. older patients may be more easily intoxicated, this factor is not usually tested in present assays. Previous chemo and radiation therapy may leave the patient altered, for example with impaired marrow reserves, or renal impairment which might make it important to test the effect of lower drug concentrations in the assay, and to develop tests which include some normal tissues in the assay by which to predict the relative effects on normal tissues and tumor.

D. The actual test procedures provide strengths, and also limitations, for specific situations. One type of assay examines the tissue of the primary tumor. Constitutive assays of fixed and stained materials have some definite predictive value for hematologic malignancies. Examinations of fresh tissues for receptors can provide predictive prognosis for later treatment with steroids and antisteroids of patients with breast, endometrial, prostate and lymphocytic tumors. Empirically, we have learned that some patients with leukemia will respond to thiopurines, but no solid tumors respond. We have also learned that bleomycin may be effective in male but not female germ cell neoplasms. Cisplatin may help non-small cell, but not small cell lung cancer. Using these concepts one can examine the fresh cells of tumors of the types known to respond, with the intent of identifying the specific patients in the responding subgroups. This might be done by looking at the tumor for pharmacologic determinants of drug effectiveness: uptake and retention of methotreate, lack of outward transport of actinomycins and anthracyclines, phosphorylation of antipurines and antipyrimidines, endogenous rates of repair of DNA damage induced by radiation and alkylating agents. In addition to tests predictive of whether the drug can be delivered to or lethally activated by the tumor cell, additional assays are currently available to examine for inactivation of drug by deamination, dephosphorylation, or hydrolysis. Assays for minimizing drug effects can be done by examining sulfhydryl, amino acid, and gluthathione tumor tissue concentrations. A large battery of tests is required for this since each drug may have a number of steps to activation and catabolism. This puts demands for more tissue or miniaturization of test samples. Also, since the final drug action is commonly to decrease tumor DNA, drug effectiveness may also require a special pathway to be present in the tumor; for example MTX and F-dump cannot be effective if the tumor uses preformed thymidine instead of deoxyuridylate for DNA synthesis. All of these tests can be done without growing the tissue, and without attempting to perturb the tumor by drug treatment. Any of these tests can predict negatively for failure more effectively than for response.

Tests which involve drug perturbations of whole tumors have the disadvantage of requiring fresh tissue, much tissue, repeated sampling and long observation times. They have the potential advantage of allowing the cell and host integrate individual drug variables because the end points are global effects on the target in the tumor and incorporate tumor cell phosphorylation, transport, binding and other single drug-oriented factors, as well as such host factors as distribution volume, plasma binding, hepatic activation (cytoxan) or destruction (cytarabine, vincas) or renal excretion (platinum, MTX).

For many tumors, short-term culture of surviving tumor cells will suffice, when DNA synthesis is the common target for many anticancer drugs, by the methods of Dr. Sylvestrini and similar techniques of Dr. Kerns. Less complicated than direct measurements of inhibition synthesis of DNA or other macromolecules in surviving cell cultures, are the more general tests of overall cytotoxicity. These are often based upon the initial observation by Schreck that cells with drug-damaged plasma membranes do not exclude dyes such as eosin added to the growth medium. Many other tests of drug induced cytotoxicity have been proposed, with end points as simple as changes in pH, and decrease in cell numbers. These tests have the problems--(1) that the end points measured are different from the targets acted on by the drug, (2) the effects may be too general, or, (3) the selection of an in vitro drug level which is higher than that tolerated in clinical situations by the normal host tissues, and (4) that in the clinical situation there may be repair of the chromosomal damage. The result is that the tests, when negative, are often accurate, but may have a high frequency of false positive prediction. Some of these problems have been sucessfully addressed by the newer modifications developed by Weisenthal and discussed later in this volume.

Somewhat more complicated are the in vitro techniques pioneered by the Toronto workers for myeloma cells, and expanded by Hamburger and others. In these tumor cells are grown in vitro in agar, and exposed for a short interval to drugs with potential antitumor effects. The end point is reduction in the amount of cell proliferation as compared to non-treatment controls. Such antiproliferative effects can be measured by counting cell numbers, or by looking for the growth of colonies over time. Many problems have

plagued this type of test, including poor growth of all but
a few types of tumors, requirement for larger numbers of
cells than can often be obtained, poor assayability of
several classes of drugs, especially the antimetabolites.
A major problem was the assumption that in vitro positivity
would correlate with clinical responsiveness, and the test
was widely advertised before careful clinical correlations
were available. A recent modification involves the use of
a special fixed matrix which appears to provide growth of
many tumors types and simplify cell counting, as reported
by Dr. Baker and colleagues in this volume. These tests
involve examination of drug-induced perturbations over
time. They come closer to the clinical situation, but lack
much ability to deal with the varying drug routes, doses,
schedules and combinations used in the clinic. Such assays
have been dubbed "clonogenic" but this is probably a
misnomer compared with "antiproliferative", since the
colonies counted have not been shown to have arisen from
single cells. It is likely that attempts to grow clones
from single cell suspensions created by the use of mechan-
ical or chemical disruption of solid tumors have added to
cell damage and failure of growth, and hence for solid
tumors a truely "clonogenic" assay would be self-defeating.

The tests most proximate to the clinical situation are
those which involve observation of drug induced changes in
tumor growth in a intact host, commonly a rodent, but also
in the intact human. The problems of accessibility for
tissues for serial sampling are formidable in humans, and
restrict such techniques to the easy serial sampling of
leukemias and malignant effusions. Serial sampling from
large tumor masses, or serial excision of multiple skin
nodules has been used in infrequent cases. Recently non-
invasive techniques have been introduced, such as external
radionuclide monitoring of intracellular uptake of labelled
drugs. Dr. Wilmann's presentation shows some of the possibilities that inhere in the study of leukemias as they are
treated with the usual doses but examined at short (days)
intervals to determine whether early changes predicted for
late (weeks) responses.

Use of animal models has been tried with varying
success over a long time. Screening with embryonated eggs
and in xenografts in hamster cheek pouches was used in new
drug selection but was not more useful than mouse ascites
tumors. Xenografts beneath the renal capsule of mice or

into nude mice have been used for new drug selection, where they are at least as effective as any other predictor for drugs which later show clinical activity. They are time-consuming and expensive, and are now being replaced, as are the ascites tumors, by the NCI cell-lines described by Dr. Handschumacher.

Of all the integrative "in vivo" or "perturbational" models, the test which comes closest to ideal, both for individualizing human treatment, and predicting effectiveness in new agents seems to be the subrenal capsular, "SRC". It permits the growth of virtually all tumors, the effective use of all drugs, and the use of a variety of dose schedules and routes and drug combinations. All of this takes place in an intact host in which toxicity can be observed. As reported by Dr. Bogden and others, the results are excellent, however, the cost is substantial and at present it has not been adopted for wide use.

One recurring problem inhibiting the more widespread use of predictive tests is the increasing use of drug combinations which are effective as first line therapy. If 75% of women with breast cancer, 80% of patients with leukemia, and 90% of patients with lymphoma respond to conventional combinations, there may not be an important role for a predictive test, since most clinicians would feel forced to use conventional therapy even if the test predicted otherwise. The need for a predictive test to select the best potential drug from amongst a group of totally new agents grows in the case of tumors of types which are treatment resistant e.g. renal cell carcinoma. However, a predictive test is mostly of value for tumors for which there are a number of single effective agents, and there are only a very few such tumors. This leaves prediction more important as a way of choosing a small number for clinical trial from a large number of new investigative agents. This reason to develop a predictive test is growing smaller because most patients are not treated with new drugs because of the recent NCI policy to deny new drugs to patients who have previously been exposed to any treatment. This suggests that the primary uses of Predictive Tests is in Preclinical New Drug Development, and in the selection of new agents for initial use in a few highly resistant tumors.

Prediction of Response to Cancer Therapy, pages 11–41
© 1988 Alan R. Liss, Inc.

IDENTIFICATION OF ENDOCRINE RESPONSIVE BREAST AND
ENDOMETRIAL CARCINOMA USING STEROID HORMONE RECEPTORS

James L. Wittliff, Thomas G. Day, Jr., William
L. Dean and Joseph C. Allegra
Departments of Biochemistry (JLW, WLD),
Obstetrics and Gynecology (TCD) and Medicine
(JCA), James Graham Brown Cancer Center,
University of Louisville, Louisville, KY 40292

I. INTRODUCTION

Normal breast is an organ in which peptide and steroid
hormonal interactions influence molecular processes
involved in proliferation, differentiation and secretion.
Although the specific role of each hormone is unknown,
estrogens, progesterone and certain glucocorticoids are
known to influence these processes. Likewise, androgen is
known to exert negative control of proliferation of breast
epithelium during early development. Several peptide
hormones such as insulin, prolactin and possibly growth
hormone and certain growth factors, in concert with the
steroid hormones, bring about the orderly differentiation
of the resting breast cell of the female to a structurally
and finally functionally, differentiated state.

The concept underlying endocrine therapy is that
certain tumor cells have retained the molecular mechanisms
(receptors) to respond to the same hormonal perturbations
as their normal progenitor cells. With specific hormone
binding data, we derive information about the natural
history of the lesion such as transformation
(dedifferentiation) which may result in the loss of
receptors and exploit their presence by employing hormone
therapy as in the case of tamoxifen administration.

Presently, both estrogen (ER) and progestin receptors
(PR) are used routinely in the clinical management of
breast and endometrial cancer as predictive indices of a
patient's response to endocrine therapy and as prognostic

indicators of a patient's clinical course (e.g. Anonymous, 1980; Wittliff, 1984; Fisher et al., 1983; Creasman et al., 1985). Clearly, this is a decade of enormous progress in the field of hormone receptors of all types. Soon additional receptor tests will be added to the oncologist's armamentarium to combat breast and other hormonally responsive neoplasia.

II. METHODS OF ANALYSES

Clinical determinations of steroid receptors are performed primarily by the multipoint titration and sucrose gradient analyses (Wittliff and Wiehle, 1985). The titration procedure is the most commonly employed and utilizes dextran-coated charcoal to remove unbound steroid from that associated with intracellular receptors.

Increasing evidence suggests steroid receptors are located in nuclei (King and Greene, 1984; Welshons et al., 1984) although the exact location in a target cell is currently debated. Receptors are soluble regulatory proteins found in cytosolic extracts of target cells. Cytosol is accepted as an operational definition referring to the soluble portion of the cell, both nuclear and cytoplasmic. Most steroid receptors are extremely labile and exist in the presence of other binding components, complicating measurements of their binding properties. Receptors associate with their particular steroid hormone in a reversible fashion and with high affinity and ligand specificity.

The rates of association and dissociation of steroid hormones with specific binding sites in cytosol from breast are dependent upon incubation time and temperature according to the reaction:

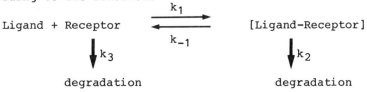

$$\text{Ligand + Receptor} \underset{k_{-1}}{\overset{k_1}{\rightleftharpoons}} \text{[Ligand-Receptor]}$$

$$\downarrow k_3 \qquad\qquad\qquad\qquad \downarrow k_2$$

$$\text{degradation} \qquad\qquad\qquad \text{degradation}$$

Loss in binding appears to be due to degradation of the receptor protein itself whether or not its binding sites are occupied by steroid. Thus, the majority of binding reactions are performed at 0-3° C.

Multipoint Titration Assay

To demonstrate the affinity and concentration of steroid receptors in a cytosol preparation, aliquots are incubated with increasing concentrations of various labeled steroids for 5-18 hours at 0-3° C. Routinely [3H]estradiol-17B and [3H]R5020 are used as labeled ligands to measure ER and PR, respectively. Recently, [125I]iodoestradiol was shown to be a highly sensitive ligand for ER and PR (Hochberg, 1979). Binding in the presence of an excess of unlabeled inhibitor is related to nonreceptor or nonspecific (low affinity, high capacity) association of the ligand. Specific association is estimated as the difference between total and nonspecific binding. The use of a double-label procedure also increases sensitivity (Grill et al., 1984).

Using Scatchard analysis, the affinity constant may be determined from the slope of the plot according to the equation:

$$\text{Slope} = 1/K_d \text{ where } K_d = 1/K_a = k_{-1}/k_1$$

Binding capacity is estimated from the intercept on the abscissa. By definition, the higher the affinity of the binding site, the lower the dissociation constant which is a measure of the tendency of the steroid-receptor complex to dissociate. The rate of this first order process is dependent upon both the type of ligand used in the assay and the kind of receptor being measured (Wittliff, 1987a). K_d values of 10^{-10} M to 10^{-11} M for ER and 10^{-9} M to 10^{-10} M for PR appearing on a patient's chart are good indicators that the biopsy contains high affinity components. Usually specific binding capacity is expressed in femtomoles (10^{-15} moles) of labeled steroid bound per mg cytosol protein (mcp).

Sucrose Density Gradient Centrifugation

Sucrose gradient centrifugation separates the various forms of the steroid receptors based upon size and shape properties (Wittliff, 1984, Wittliff and Wiehle, 1985).

Using this method, we showed the sedimentation profiles of either ER or PR in human breast carcinomas fall into four general categories. These are tumors which contain receptors migrating at either 8S (Svedbergs) only, 4S only or both 8S and 4S and those in which receptors are undetectable. The sedimentation coefficients of 8S and 4S are only approximate and are used operationally. The majority of breast tumors containing ER exhibit both the 8S and 4S isoforms. Ten to fifteen percent of biopsies contained only the 4S species using sucrose gradient centrifugation with conditions of low ionic strength (Wittliff et al., 1978). Our laboratory has suggested this receptor polymorphism has clinical significance (Wittliff, 1984).

High Performance Liquid Chromatography

Steroid receptors are dynamic proteins whose properties of size, shape, surface charge, and hydrophobicity vary depending on the conditions of their environment. Using various types of chromatography, one can exploit these properties so that the various species (isoforms) of the receptors can be separated (Wittliff, 1986).

To circumvent the problems associated with prolonged manipulation of receptor preparations such as proteolysis or ligand dissociation, the use of high-performance liquid chromatography (HPLC) in size exclusion, ion exchange, chromatofocusing, and hydrophobic interaction modes was developed for rapid, effective separation of receptor isoforms (Wittliff and Wiehle, 1985, Wittliff, 1986). HPLC separation has shown that receptors exhibit polymorphism. This is an indication that their composition is far more complicated than originally assumed. We suggested the use of the term "fractionated receptors" to designate the pattern of the various steroid hormone-binding components (isoforms) displayed by a single receptor type.

A representative profile of ER isoforms separated based on surface charge properties using high performance chromatofocusing is shown in Figure 1. The clinical significance of isoform profiles is currently the subject of considerable research in our group. We have learned that various physiological conditions appear to alter the relative amounts and distribution of ER and PR isoforms.

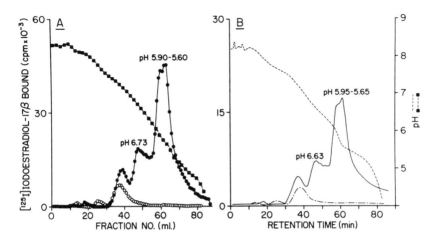

Figure 1. HPCF separation of ionic isoforms of ER from breast cancer. [125I]iodoestradiol in the absence (●) and presence (O) of unlabeled diethylstilbestrol was used as ligand. The profiles in A were generated by manual counting while that shown in B was made with an on-line radioisotope detector (taken from Boyle et al, 1985).

Some of these parameters include patient age, endocrine status, and history of therapeutic manipulation (Wittliff, 1987a). Application of "fractionated receptor" profiles to clinical management of breast cancer must await additional investigation.

Monoclonal Antibody Based Assays

Most immunohistochemical techniques for localization of receptors utilize highly specific monoclonal antibodies (MAb) directed against the partially purified receptor (e.g. Greene et al., 1980). Sections from a freshly frozen biopsy are required. A peroxidase-antiperoxidase method for immunocytochemical staining is employed giving a largely qualitative estimate. The procedure is primarily for investigational use and is being correlated with conventional ligand-binding assays (King et al., 1985; McCarty et al., 1985). It is unclear whether these MAb react with the various isoforms of ER to the same extent (Sato et al., 1986).

The enzyme-linked immunochemical assay is also based on a sandwich technique that involves two specific MAb prepared against the partially purified ER (Greene et al., 1980, King et al., 1984). The first antibody (D-547) which is immobilized on a polystyrene bead, is incubated with cytosol prepared in buffer. After incubation and complexing of ER with MAb, the bead is washed and a second MAb(H222) that has been previously labeled with peroxidase is added. The peroxidase linked to the second MAb serves as a marker for the presence of steroid receptor. This procedure measures receptor mass in contrast to radioligand-binding techniques, which measure the steroid-binding capacity. However, most workers relate EIA results to binding capacity expressed as fmol/mcp. There appears to be considerable variation in ER levels measured by the titration assay compared to that observed with the EIA (Mirecki and Jordan, 1985; Anonymous, 1986, Raam and Vrabel, 1986) with a greater receptor level by the EIA method. Since the molecular basis of this difference is unclear, the assay is still under investigation.

III. REFERENCE RANGES AND DISTRIBUTION

Breast Cancer

Generally, >3 fmol/mcp represents an ER level correlated with the lack of response of a breast cancer patient given endocrine therapy of either the ablative or additive type (Anonymous, 1980). Although there is a "borderline" range of 3 to 10 or 20 fmol/mcp, binding capacities of >10 fmol ER appear to represent clinically significant levels as shown by the NSABP (Fisher et al., 1983). We have observed values of more than 5000 fmol/mcp for ER and 6000 fmol/mcp for PR in certain tumors (Table 1). ER levels in biopsies from premenopausal patients appear considerably lower than those of postmenopausal women with breast carcinoma. In general, a higher PR was observed in biopsies from both pre- and post-menopausal women when ER was present also (Wittliff, 1984). However, a lower PR level was measured in the absence of ER, supporting the suggestion that the formation of the latter receptor is dependent upon estrogen action (Horwitz et al., 1975).

TABLE 1. Specific Binding Capacities of Steroid Receptors in Breast Tumor Biopsies According to Patient Endocrine Status[a]

Steroid Receptor Level (fmol/mg protein)[b]		Endocrine Status of Patient	Receptor Status of Tumor
Estrogen	Progestin		
89 ± 9 (10-1335)	238 ± 22 (10-3038)	Premenopausal	ER^+/PR^+
83 ± 15 (10-568)	---	Premenopausal	ER^+/PR^-
---	84 ± 18 (10-1151)	Premenopausal	ER^-/PR^+
286 ± 18 (10-5693)	336 ± 28 (10-5922)	Postmenopausal	ER^+/PR^+
176 ± 29 (10-2807)	---	Postmenopausal	ER^+/PR^-
---	75 ± 26 (10-977)	Postmenopausal	ER^-/PR^+

[a]Adapted from Bland et al. (1981).
[b]>10 fmol/mg cytosol protein taken as an arbitrary "cut-off" value as utilized by the NSABP.

The multipoint titration assay is a reference standard for all new receptor methods. Since this assay has been used in the authors' laboratory for thousands of breast cancer biopsies, reference ranges are well defined (Wittliff, 1987a,b,). Specific binding capacity is influenced by menopausal status indicating reference ranges should be considered in terms of this factor. Table 2 provides an example of the distribution of ER and according to endocrine status. Kd values of 10^{-10} to ^{11}M are representative of ER and PR.

A number of other clinical factors influencing steroid binding capacity include sex, age, day of cycle in premenopausal patients, pregnancy and lactation and previous drug administration. The curious distribution in which ER is lacking and PR is present is seen three times more often in biopsies of premenopausal patients than in the postmenopausal patients (Table 2). This appears to be due to the presence of circulating estrogens in the plasma masking the steroid hormone receptors in a tumor biopsy (Wittliff, 1984).

TABLE 2. Distribution of Steroid Receptors in Tumor Biopsies According to Patient Endocrine Status[a]

	Endocrine Status of Patient	
Receptor Status	Premenopausal	Postmenopausal
ER$^+$/PR$^+$	222 (45%)	520 (63%)
ER$^+$/PR$^-$	58 (12%)	128 (15%)
ER$^-$/PR$^-$	136 (28%)	137 (17%)
ER$^-$/PR$^+$	72 (15%)	41 (5%)

[a]Results related to assays described in Table 1 (adapted from Bland et al., 1981).

Endogenous hormones or hormonal-like drugs such as tamoxifen and medroxyprogesterone bind readily to ER and PR respectively and associate tightly with the nuclear components (matrix and chromatin). Since they may influence the actual levels of receptors in a target cell leading to altered radio-ligand binding values, knowledge of previous therapy of a patient is essential.

Endometrial Cancer

Endometrial cancer occurs in the presence of a target cell population exhibiting steroid hormone sensitivity. This is unlike breast cancer in which the tumor arises in epithelial cells among a population composed primarily of connective tissue and adipose cells lacking steroid hormone receptors. Therefore, to define the ranges for endometrial cancer, one must consider the ER and PR levels in normal uterus as a useful reference.

Figure 2 provides a representative distribution of ER and PR in uteri from women with no evidence of uterine cancer. In addition to a population of biopsies containing both receptors as expected, there was a small population of normal uteri that contained only PR (Van der Walt et al., 1986). This is in distinction to the accepted hypothesis that the ER is necessary for PR formation (Horwitz et al., 1975). We postulated from these data and other information that there may be a constitutive isoform which is influenced very little by the estrogen concentration and a

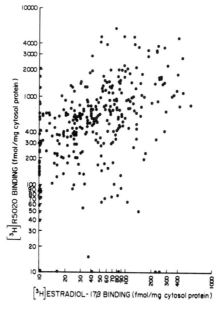

Figure 2 The relationship between PR levels and the corresponding ER levels in 319 human uteri. Taken from van der Walt et al., 1986

second type which is under the control of estrogen and possibly other hormonal factors (van der Walt et al., 1986).

ER in normal uteri ranged from undetectable to 560 fmol/mcp while that of PR ranged from undetectable to > 5000 fmol/mcp using the multipoint titration assay. In contrast, the reference ranges for endometrial cancer were from undetectable to 611 fmol/mcp ER and from undetectable to 3647 fmol/mcp (Fuchs et al, 1987). The mean ER level of 131 biopsies was 45 ± 97 fmol/mcp ($K_d = 2 \pm 4 \times 10^{-10}$M) and that of PR was 104 ± 260 fmol/mcp ($K_d = 4 \pm 7 \times 10^{-10}$M) using the multipoint titration assay. Unlike normal uterus, many biopsies of uterine cancer do not contain either of these receptors. Our personal experience is that 38% of these tumors do not contain either receptor while 39% contained both types. Eight percent of endometrial cancers contained only the PR and 15% contained only ER.

The mean K_d value for the ER was 4×10^{-10} M while that for the PR was 9.2×10^{-10} M from analyses of 319 noncancerous human uteri. It is generally accepted that K_d values of the ER and PR in normal and cancerous uteri are similar to those reported in breast cancer. We highly recommend that an individual laboratory develop its own distribution profiles of steroid hormone receptors such as presented in Figure 2 including the levels found in the various types of tumors. These should be compared with studies published in the literature to insure that a laboratory is generating comparable information, thus indicating a valid procedure.

IV. QUALITY ASSURANCE

Since the procedures and various programs for establishing uniformity of steroid receptors have been described elsewhere (e.g. Sarfaty et al., 1981; Wittliff et al., 1981) they are mentioned briefly. As a result of reports presented at the First International Workshop on Estrogen Receptors in Breast Cancer (McGuire et al., 1975), it was obvious that greater efforts must be made to establish uniformity and quality control of receptor methods. In fact, one of the conclusions drawn from the 1979 NIH Consensus Development Conference (Anonymous, 1980) was that "there is a need for quality control of steroid receptor assays." Since 1977, the Hormone Receptor Laboratory at the University of Louisville has established a reference facility for monitoring quality assurance of steroid receptors in biopsies of breast and endometrial carcinomas.

Each shipment of reference powders is designed according to the specific need of the cooperative trial groups and shipped on dry ice to the participating laboratories. Thus far, our laboratory has cooperated with the National Surgical Breast and Bowel Adjuvant Project (NSABP), Southeastern Cancer Study Group, Southwest Oncology Group, Cancer and Leukemia Group B, North Central Cancer Treatment Group and the Eastern Cooperative Oncology Group. We also collaborate with the College of American Pathologists in providing annual surveys. Currently, we have assisted more than 350 laboratories in North America and have worked with various laboratories in Europe, South America, Asia, Australia, and Africa to establish quality assurance measures.

It is essential that a laboratory utilize a daily quality control material and periodically participate in an outside quality assurance program such as those established by the clinical cooperative groups. Criteria for evaluating agreement of results are to be established by committees composed of oncologists and clinical chemists. The committee contacts each laboratory in writing regarding their performance relative to that of the reference laboratory and other laboratories taking part in the clinical trial. This important information should be available to the physician treating the patient. In this way, meaningful relationships between biochemical markers such as the steroid hormone receptors and clinical response to experimental therapies can be realized.

V. CLINICAL STUDIES

Breast Cancer

If the hypothesis (Horwitz et al., 1975) is correct that the presence of functional ER is required for the formation of PR, there should be a direct relationship between these two receptors in responsive cells. The majority of the breast tumors containing both receptors would be assumed to retain hormonal responsiveness. A summary of results presented at the Consensus Development Conference (Anonymous, 1980) is shown in Table 3. From measurements of receptor status of each tumor biopsy, 78% of patients with breast tumors containing both receptors responded objectively to hormone therapy. If only ER was present, a 34% response rate was observed while only 10% of patients responded to endocrine manipulation if neither receptor was present in the breast tumor. In North America this value drops to 3%, possibly due to increased emphasis on qualaity assurance programs (Wittliff et al., 1981). Surprisingly, 5 of 11 patients responded objectively to hormone therapy, although each had breast tumors containing only the PR. This appears puzzling if there is a relationship between ER and PR in responsive tumors and may be related to the endocrine status of the patient. These latter data suggest that the progestin receptor may be particularly important in the selection of premenopausal patients for endocrine manipulation (Bland et al., 1981). Clark et al. (1983) also showed PR was a strong prognostic index.

TABLE 3. Relationship Between Steroid-Receptor Status of Breast Tumor and Patient's Objective Response to Endocrine Therapy[a]

Steroid Receptor Status[b]			
ER+/PR+	ER+/PR−	ER−/PR−	ER−/PR+
135/174 (78%)	55/164 (34%)	17/165 (10%)	5/11 (45%)

[a]NIH Consensus Development Conference on Steroid Receptors in Breast Cancer, 1979 (Anonymous, 1980).
[b]Ratio of number of patients responding to number with receptor status designated.

The NSABP initiated a prospectively randomized clinical trial for women with primary operable breast cancer and positive axillary nodes in 1977. 1891 patients were randomized to receive L-phenylalanine mustard and 5-flurouracil (PF) either with or without tamoxifen (T). In this interim report the median follow-up time was 3 yr (Fisher et al., 1983). Patients >50 yr of age with either 1-3 or >3 positive axillary nodes had a markedly longer disease-free survival on PFT than those receiving PF adjuvant therapy. The effectiveness of PFT was related to tumor levels of steroid receptors. Patients >50 yr old with both tumor ER and PR levels of >10 fmole displayed the greatest benefit in disease-free survival from PFT. Patients <50 yr with tumor ER and PR levels <10 fmole had a poorer survival when given PFT. Those whose tumors demonstrated a high ER and a low PR also had a shorter survival on PFT. The observation of no benefit in younger patients when both receptor levels were high, but a benefit in older patients with receptor-poor tumors, indicates that the difference between the two age groups cannot be explained by the association of age with receptor content under the conditions of this study (Fisher et al., 1983). Multivariate analyses supported the conclusion that, while nodes and ER exerted strong prognostic influences in both PF and PFT-treated patients, the PR content of tumors was a stronger predictor of the effectiveness of PFT therapy than was ER content. This suggested a heterogeneity in response to PFT therapy that was both age and PR dependent. The findings emphasized the need for accurate quantative determinations of both the ER and PR content of tumors. The data indicated that T should not be administered with PF to patients under 60 yr of age with PR-poor tumors and finally they suggested that prolonged administration of T may be clinically useful (Fisher et al., 1983).

For many years, hormonal therapy has been the mainstay of the early treatment of Stage IV breast cancer. Endocrine manipulations lead to 50-60% response rates in women with ER+ tumors with prolonged survival and a good quality of life. Cytotoxic chemotherapy yields equivalent response rates with acceptable toxicity and is an excellent means of palliation especially of hormone-independent tumors which do not respond to hormone therapy. However with either treatment most all remissions are partial responses.

One aspect of tumor biology which is likely to be involved in our inability to attain complete remissions in breast cancer is cellular heterogeneity. It is known that

ER positive tumors are composed predominantly of ER^+ cells, but also contain cells which lack these receptors. Likewise, ER^- tumors contain primary cells lacking ER although a few cells possess ER. To attack these divergent populations of cells, recent clinical investigators have empirically designed combinations of hormone therapy and chemotherapy aimed at killing the ER^+ component and the rapidly dividing ER^- component of the tumor. Thus far, combination chemo-hormonal therapy regimens have yielded slightly higher overall remission rates, but no significant increase in complete remissions.

A Phase II clinical trial was designed to test a variant of standard combination chemo-hormonal therapy, i.e. synchronization - stimulation of tumor cells in order to potentially increase the chemo-responsiveness of breast cancer (Allegra et al., 1982). In this concept, endocrine therapy is utilized to synchronize tumor cells then rescue by a second hormonal manipulation. The rescue aspect of this schema is an attempt to increase the number of cells in the S phase of the cell cycle similar to cell culture studies described by Lippman et al.(1976, 1984). The cells are then subsequently treated with S phase-specific cytotoxic chemotherapy in an attempt to further enhance cell kill.

The combination chemo-hormonal therapy schema in Figure 3 is based upon the observations that breast cancers exhibit cellular heterogeneity with regard to ER and that hormonal and chemotherapy have different mechanisms of action and of toxicity, and further that cell cycle specific agents are most effective against rapidly dividing cells. Our hypothesis (Allegra et al., 1982) was that utilizing hormones and chemotherapy in this manner would result in a better response when compared to either therapy alone.

Thirty of the patients, or 53%, had tumors which were ER^+. Twenty were ER^-, and 7 had tumors of unknown ER status. All receptor assays were performed using assays meeting compliance criteria (Wittliff et al., 1981). A cutoff value for positivity of 10 fmol/mcp was chosen.

Fifty-seven patients were entered into this Phase II clinical trial. All were evaluable for response, survival and toxicity. Thirty-eight of the patients (67%) have one

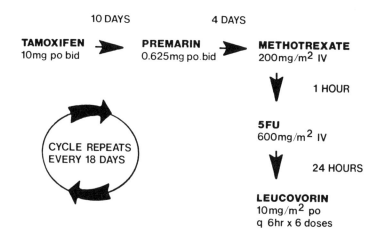

Figure 3. Synchronization-stimulation of metastatic breast cancer using combination hormonal-chemotherapy.

site of metastatic disease; 15 patients (26%) had two sites involved with metastatic tumor and only four patients had three or more sites of metastases. Approximately, 25% of patients had either bone or visceral dominant disease while 50% of patients had soft tissue dominant disease.

Overall response rate was 62% with 37% complete remissions and 25% partial remissions (Allegra et al., 1987). Stable disease was achieved in 21% of patients and only 17% of patients exhibited progressive disease on this regimen. There were no significant differences in response as a function of ER status (ER[+] 70%, ER unknown 71%, ER[-] 45%), menopausal status (pre-65%, post-50%), dominate site of disease (bone - 50%, soft tissue - 66%, visceral - 64%) or prior therapy (none - 71%, prior RT - 59%, prior chemo- 50%, prior hormones - 50%).

The median duration of remission was 14 months. The median survival for the responders was 28 mo and 14 mo for the non-responders. This two-fold increase in median survival was significant (P<0.01). A larger patient population with both ER and PR levels on biopsies is required to fully ascertain the role of sex-steroid receptors in synchronization-stimulation therapy of metastatic breast cancer.

Endometrial Cancer

Progestin administration has been used routinely in the treatment of endometial carcinoma with a <30% response rate. To improve patient selection, a number of studies have shown that PR content correlates well with response to progestin therapy (e.g. Creasman et al., 1980; Erhlich et al., 1981; Kauppila et al., 1982). More recently Martin et al (1983) demonstrated increased survival of patients with ER+ uterine cancer. Perhaps the most comprehensive study has been that of Creasman et al., (1985) who reported that ER, PR as well as combined ER/PR status were significant independent prognostic factors, replacing histologic assessment of glandular or nuclear differentiation. Thus, ER and PR content of endometrial cancer permits an improved prediction of prognosis and appears helpful in predicting responses to therapy at the time of a future recurrence. Furthermore, these and other studies provided a basis for examining the use of antiestrogen and progestin therapies in uterine carcinoma.

Hormonal Recruitment Therapy

A pilot study conducted by Swenerton et al. (1979) to assess the efficacy of tamoxifen in advanced endometrial carcinoma demonstrated response in four of several eluable patients. These preliminary data suggested that patients with lower-grade tumors and longer disease-free intervals were more likely to respond than those with higher-grade tumors and shorter disease-free intervals. Furthermore, there was a suggestion that cross-resistance did not occur between progestins and tamoxifen. Also, such treatment showed remarkably little toxicity, a particular advantage in a group of patients who are often elderly and whose coexistent illness makes them unsuitable for intensive combination chemotherapy. Finally, Mortel et al. (1981) reported that short-term administration of the antiestrogen, tamoxifen, led to increased PR in 11 of 15 endometial carcinomas including 4 which were initially PR⁻. The ability of tamoxifen to increase PR via the antiestrogen mechanism coupled with its low cytotoxicity makes the combination of tamoxifen with a progestational agent a scientifically sound therapeutic approach. Operationally we have described hormonal recruitment therapy as the use of hormone-related drugs or anti-hormones to recruit (induce) cells to a therapeutically sensitive state.

Our hypothesis was that sustained or intermittent use of tamoxifen 1) induces PR in tumors, 2) increases the duration of response to progestin therapy by hormonally sensitive tumors and 3) increases the absolute number of progestin responsive patients by induction of PR in tumors which were initially PR⁻. The treatment protocol is shown in Figure 4 (Carlson et al., 1984). Thus far 54 patients have been treated. An example of tamoxifen's influence on ER and PR is shown in Table 4. Note that in addition to the induction of PR in most grade 2 carcinomas, tamoxifen occasionally increased ER to very high levels. As shown in Table 5, tamoxifen increased the incidence of PR from 48% to 80% indicating this aspect of our hypothesis was correct. As expected short-term tamoxifen administration decreased ER incidence from 54% to 41% after 5 days of therapy. Since the trial is on going, clinical response data are still being collected. Our study suggests tamoxifen improves the candidacy of many patients for progestin treatment who previously would have been given non-hormonal therapies.

VI. A NEW MARKER FOR PREDICTING TAMOXIFEN-UNRESPONSIVE BREAST CANCERS WHICH ARE ER⁺

Our long term goal is to determine if cytochrome P-450 plays a role in responsiveness of human breast and endometrial carcinomas to additive endocrine therapy (Fig.5).

It is known that liver microsomal cytochrome P-450 is involved in steroid metabolism and probably also participates in the metabolism of anti-estrogens such as tamoxifen (Jordan, 1985). In mammals, cytochrome P-450 linked enzymes are present in the endoplasmic reticulum

Figure 4. Combination hormonal therapy in advanced tamoxifen (Jordan, 1985). In mammals, cytochrome P-450 endometrial carcinoma.

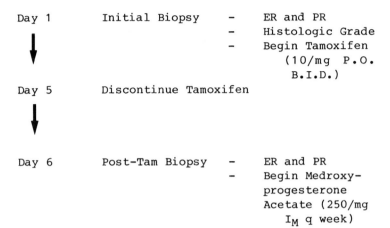

Day 1	Initial Biopsy	–	ER and PR
		–	Histologic Grade
		–	Begin Tamoxifen (10/mg P.O. B.I.D.)
Day 5	Discontinue Tamoxifen		
Day 6	Post-Tam Biopsy	–	ER and PR
		–	Begin Medroxy-progesterone Acetate (250/mg I_M q week)

TABLE 4. Alterations in Estrogen and Progesterone Receptors in Histologic Grade 2 Endometrial Carcinoma After Tamoxifen

Progesterone receptors (fmol/mg cyt. prot.)		Estrogen receptors (fmol/mg cyt. prot.)	
Initial biopsy	Biopsy after tamoxifen	Initial biopsy	Biopsy after tamoxifen
316	1242	182	7405
UD	15	UD	714
UD	57	8	UD
14	306	14	UD
40	1415	38	19
UD	40	UD	UD
28	138	67	20
63	88	58	4
10	134	UD	UD
137	35	71	27
2293	638	258	114

TABLE 5. Tamoxifen Induction of Progestin Receptors in Endometrial Carcinoma

Treatment	Receptor Presence (>10 fmol/mcp)	
	Progestin	Estrogen
Pre-Tamoxifen	26/54 (48%)	29/54 (54%)
Post-Tamoxifen	43/54 (80%)	22/54 (41%)

at varying concentrations in almost all tissues. However, very little research has been performed concerning the existence and role of cytochrome P-450 in normal and neoplastic reproductive tissues. Furthermore, the probable involvement of cytochrome P-450 in breast or uterine carcinogenesis, either by converting procarcinogens into carcinogens, local metabolism of chemotherapeutic drugs or estrogen synthesis remained to be demonstrated in these tissues.

It is possible that variations in cytochrome P-450 levels in human breast and endometrial carcinomas may influence their responsiveness to endocrine therapy (Fig. 5). Therefore a simple sensitive spectrophotometic assay for determining levels of cytochrome P-450-dependent cyclohexane hydroxylation activity in breast and uterine microsomes was developed (Senler et al., 1985a). Cyclohexane was chosen as a substrate because of the relatively high levels of cyclohexane hydroxylase activity in tumor microsomes and because cyclohexane serves as a substrate for several forms of cytochrome P-450. A direct method utilizing isotope-dilution/gas chromatography-mass spectrometry was also developed in order to confirm the results of the spectrophotometric assay. The average activity (cyclohexane-dependent NADPH oxidation) for 139 human breast-tumor microsome preparations was 1.34 nmol/min/mg which is in the range of that found in untreated mammalian liver (1-3/nmol/min/mg). Also, high enzyme activity was demonstrated in human ovary, normal uterus as well as uterine leiomyomas. Endocrine status appeared to influence enzyme levels, in that mammary tissue from virgin rats contained significantly higher amounts of activity than did tissues from either pregnant or lactating rats. Furthermore, carbon monoxide, as well as an antibody against rat liver cytochrome P-450, completely inhibited

NADPH oxidation by breast-carcinoma microsomes. These results strengthen our hypothesis that tumors with high levels of cytochrome P-450 may have a reduced response to additive endocrine therapy.

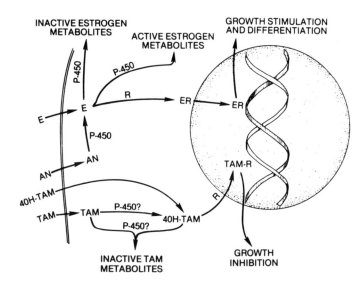

Figure 5. Possible interactions of sex-steroid hormones and antihormones in a target cell.

To examine the role of cytochrome P-450 in breast cancer, enzyme levels were evaluated as related to established markers of endocrine response, i.e. ER and PR levels (Senler et al., 1985b). There was no apparent correlation between cyclohexane hydroxylation activity and ER and/or PR levels. When receptor status of the individual breast tumor was compared, there was no significant difference in enzyme activity between women with ER+/PR+ and ER-/PR- tumors (Fig. 6). Furthermore, no significant difference in enzyme activity was observed in breast tumor microsomes between premenopausal and postmenopausal women. Also, there was no significant difference for both premenopausal and postmenopausal women who were each separately categorized into ER+/PR+ and ER-/PR- tumors. However, 9 of 31 (29%) tumors from premenopausal women contained greater than 1000 pmol/min/mg cytochrome P-450 dependent hydroxylation activity while 38 of 80 (48%) tumors from postmenopausal patients exhibited at least these levels. Thus, both groups contained a significant number of patients with enzyme activity levels in the range of mammalian liver.

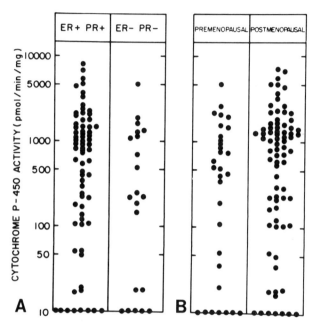

Figure 6. Relationship between cyclohexan hydoxylation activity and patient endocrine status in human breast cancer.

A. Breast tumors with ER and PR levels of >10 fmol/mcp were categorized as positive (70) and those below 10 fmol/mcp were considered negative (21). The mean ± S.E. of hydroxylation activity (pmol/min/mg) for the ER+/PR+ group (1505 ± 215) was not significantly different (p>.05) from the ER⁻/PR⁻ group (905 ± 278)

B. Breast tumors from women >55 yr of age were categorized as postmenopausal (80) and those under 55 yr were considered premenopausal (31). The mean ± S.E. of cyclohexane-dependent NADPH oxidation (pmol/min/mg) from the postmenopausal group (1534 ± 193) was not significantly different (p>.05) from women in the premenopausal group (1004 ± 230). Cyclohexane hydroxylation activity of 10 pmol/min/mg or less were scored as 10 for both studies (A & B). Taken from Senler et al., 1985b.

Cytochrome P-450 biosynthesis did not appear to be regulated either by ER or PR since no correlation was found between receptor levels and enzyme activity. However, this is not to imply that there is no relationship between these two activities in a given breast tumor from the standpoint of a patient's response to additive hormone therapy. For instance, a significant number of tumors had high levels of both ER/PR and enzyme activity.

It is now widely accepted that receptor determinations are useful in selecting patients for chemotherapy or hormone therapy (Wittliff, 1984). However, in a significant fraction (approximately 40%) of patients whose tumors exhibit ER with or without PR (Table 3) no response to endocrine therapy was observed. We have suggestged that this lack of response may be due to "defective" ER in certain tumors (Wittliff et al., 1978). Based on results of this study, it is also possible that women with breast tumors containing ER and high cytochrome P-450 activity may be less responsive to therapies utilizing tamoxifen or other hormonal agents by metabolizing them to inactive metabolites. Thus, the ER mechanism would be rendered ineffective. Future considerations should include testing this hypothesis by analyzing patient response to administrative endocrine therapy and correlating this with cytochrome P-450 activities in breast cancer.

VII. RECEPTOR POLYMORPHISM

The origin and physiological significance of the multiple forms of receptors have been a major focus of our investigations (Wittliff, 1984, 1986). Although certain of these components may represent distinct physiologic species, a few may arise due to proteolytic cleavage. Presumable, the latter possibility may occur during homogenization, prolonged incubation, and overnight centrifugation. To our knowledge, no one has provided conclusive evidence of the "native state" of estrogen (ER) and progestin (PR) in breast and endometrial carcinomas.

To circumvent the problem of prolonged manipulation of receptor preparations, we developed the use of high performance liquid chromatography in size exclusion (HPSEC), ion-exchange (HPIEC), chromatofocusing (HPCF) and hydrophobic interaction (HPHIC) modes for the rapid separation of isoforms (Wittliff and Wiehle, 1986; Wittliff, 1986). Receptor isoforms are defined as protein components in a target organ which exhibit a high ligand binding affinity and specificity for a single class of steroid hormone (e.g. estrogens) and may be identified based upon characteristic of size, shape and surface ionic properties.

HPLC Methods

Currently, we employ an Altex (Beckman) HPLC system with extensive flow-through detection equipment for the following measurements: UV-visible absorbance (Altex or Hitachi), conductivity (Bio-Rad), pH (Pharmacia) and gamma radioactivity (Altex). Due to the thermal lability of receptor proteins the system was installed in a temperature-controlled chromatographic chamber (Puffer Hubbard). Optimizing a mode of analysis requires attention to the characteristics of the column employed, especially the pore size, hydrophobicity, and loading capacity. Details of the various separation modes are given in recent papers (Wittliff and Wiehle, 1986; Wittliff, 1986).

Results

Table 6 provides a summary of results from our experience with ER from 5 different target organs. Note that a large molecular weight species (60-70A) was detected by HPSEC. Kinetics of its ligand binding and separation profile suggest this isoform may represent a precursor or aggregate of the receptor. A similar isoform of the PR was observed by HPSEC.

At least two charge isoforms of the ER were detected by HPIEC and HPCF. However, human uteri often exhibited 4 different isoforms by HPCF which shifted to highly acidic species with 10 mM sodium molybdate. When either [^{3}H]tamoxifen or [^{3}H]tamoxifen-40H was substituted as a ligand for the ER of rat uterus, two isoforms ware detected at 90 mM and 150 mM phosphate by HPIEC. PR exhibited one species primarily when separated by HPIEC or HPCF (Table 7) using either [^{3}H]R5020 or [^{3}H]Org-2058.

TABLE 6. Comparison of Properties of Estrogen Receptors Separated by HPLC

Tissue	HPSEC (TSK-3000 SW)	HPIEC (AX-1000)	HPCF (AX-500)
MCF-7 Cells	68 A	55 and 180 mM phosphate	pH 6.3 and 4.3
Human Breast Carcinoma	>61 A and 29-32 A	52, 100, 190 mM phosphate	pH 6.3, 5.3 4.8-3.5 shoulder
Human Uterus	>61 A and 29-32 A	115 and 203 mM phosphate	pH 7.1, 6.6 6.15 and 5.3
Rabbit Endometrial Carcinoma	71 A	50 and 175 mM phosphate	pH 6.8, 6.4 and 5.6
Rat Lactating Mammary Gland	>61 A	90 and 205 mM phosphate	pH 6.8 and 6.5

TABLE 7: Summary of Properties of Progestin Receptors in Human Uterus

Ligand	HPSEC(TSK3000 SW)	HPIEC (AX-100)	HPCF (AX500)
R5020	>80 A 35 A	100 mM phosphate	pH 5.7
ORG-2058	70 A 20 A	100 mM phosphate	pH 5.0

Summary

HPLC offers speed of analyses, sensitivity and high recoveries. Technical advancements such as synthesis of [^{125}I]iodine-labeled ligands of high specific radioactivity coupled with efficient flow-through detectors have facilitated our investigations of the properties of steroid hormone receptors. Factors we have found which may alter the profile of steroid receptor isoforms are stage of differentiation, endocrine status, age, tissue of origin, disease and administration of hormones or drugs.

Some of the cellular events which may give rise to receptor heterogeneity include proteolysis, phosphorylation, protein-protein interaction and protein-nucleic acid interaction. Regarding proteolysis, receptor isoforms may be generated by proteases released during homogenization. Another possibility is the processing of a high molecular weight precursor of the receptor which is an example of a physiologic event common in biology. Interchange between active and inactive receptor states may be modulated by phosphorylation or other post-translational modification. Other means of deriving receptor isoforms could occur either due to aggregation during extraction or via association/dissociation of receptor subunits. While the latter represents examples of protein-protein interactions, it is possible that receptor-nucleic acid complexes may also be identified in tissue preparations. Our data suggest that the level of receptor organization and interrelationships are more complicated than thought previously.

VIII. CONCLUSIONS AND RECOMMENDATIONS

Analyses of steroid receptors are important predictive tests for the identification of the individual with breast or endometrial cancer most likely to respond to hormonal therapy (Wittliff, 1984, 1987a,b). Steroid hormone receptors are considered with clinical factors such as previous response to hormone therapy, disease-free interval, age and menopausal status, and location of the dominant metastatic lesion as the principal criteria for selecting therapeutic regimens for these women. Since the original report of Folca and co-workers in 1961 indicating a greater uptake of labeled hexestrol by breast tumors of patients showing a response to ablative therapy, numerous studies have shown that approximately one-half of all biopsies of malignant breast tumors contained ER (Anonymous 1980). Furthermore, 55-60% of the patients exhibiting ER were responsive to either administrative or ablative hormone therapies. The use of this single biochemical criterion by the physician has increased by two- or three-fold, the accuracy of selecting the patient with advanced breast cancer or endometrial carcinoma most likely to respond objectively to endocrine manipulation.

In general, when ER was present, a higher PR was observed in tumor biopsies from both pre- and post-menopausal women. However, in the absence of ER, a lower

PR level was measured supporting the suggestion that the formation of the latter receptor is dependent upon estrogen action. Similar values have been reported for biopsies of endometrial cancer. Progress during the last 15 years has shown that:

- 55% to 65% of primary breast tumors contain more than 10 fmol/mg cytosol protein of ER.
- 45% to 55% of metastatic breast tumors contain more than 10 fmol/mg cytosol protein of ER.
- ER are present more often in breast tumors of postmenopausal women compared to those of premenopausal women.
- benign breast lesions such as fibrocystic disease and fibroadenomas usually contain less than 10 fmol/mcp ER.
- 90% of male breast carcinomas contain ER and less than 50% contain PR.
- approximately 55% of women with breast tumors containing ER respond objectively to endocrine therapy, either additive or ablative.
- less than 3% of women with breast tumors lacking ER respond objectively to hormone therapy.
- 45% to 60% of primary or metastatic breast tumors contain PR.
- the presence of both ER and PR in a breast tumor indicates a 75% to 80% likelihood that the patient will respond to endocrine manipulation, either additive or ablative.
- it has been suggested that the presence of 8 Svedberg isoforms of the ER and PR in a breast tumor (as detected by sucrose gradient centrifugation) improves the accuracy of selecting the patient likely to respond to endocrine therapy. The clinical significance (or rather insignificance) of the 4 S isoform of these receptors is debated currently
- both ER and PR exhibit polymorphism (presence of multiple isoforms) based upon separation and characterization using their properties of size, shape, surface ionic charge and hydrophobicity employing techniques such as high performance liquid chromatography.
- there appears to be a relationship between the quantity of both ER and PR in a breast tumor and a patient's response to endocrine therapy. The incidence of response to hormone therapy increases with increasing receptor levels.

It is recommended that both ER and PR analyses be

performed on all biopsies from patients with confirmed or suspected cases of breast and endometrial carcinoma prior to therapeutic manipulation. Use laboratories participating in quality assurance programs to establish uniformity of methods and data expression for these receptors. Receptor data (both quantitative and qualitative) may be used as (a) predictive indicators of an endocrine responsive tumor and (b) prognostic indices of a patient's clinical course. Higher levels of these receptors in a tumor biopsy are associated with a greater probability of disease-free survival. Receptor profiles (i.e. the presence of different types of receptors including those for androgen, glucocorticoid and other hormones) may be useful in the diagnosis of certain neoplasms.

IX. ACKNOWLEDGEMENTS

Studies in the Hormone Receptor Laboratory during the past decade have been supported in part by grants from the American Cancer Society (BC-514B), Phi Beta Psi Sorority, USPHS grants CA-19657, CA-34211, CA-32102, CA-37429, CA-25224, CA-42154 and CA-31946 from the National Cancer Institute and by the College of American Pathologists. We're especially appreciative of the efforts of Ms. Linda Hix and Linda Sanders in the preparation of the typescript.

X. REFERENCES

Allegra JC, Woodcock TM, Richman SP, Bland KI, Wittliff JL(1982). A phase II trial of tamoxifen, premarin, methotrexate and 5-fluorouracil in metastatic breast cancer. Breast Cancer Res. & Treatment 2:93-99.

Allegra JC, Barrows GH, Wittliff JL, Allegra MD, Kubota TK, Woodcock TM, Richard SP, Blumenreich MS, Gentile P (1987). Synchronization-stimulation of metastic breast cancer with tamoxifen, premarin, methotrexate, and 5 flourouracil." In press.

Anonymous (1980). NIH consensus development conference on steroid receptors in breast cancer. Cancer 46(12): 2759 -2963.

Anonymous (1986). Symposium on estrogen receptor determination with monoclonal Antibodies, Cancer Res 46 (Suppl 1):4231S-4314S.

Bland, KL, Fuchs A, Wittliff JL (1981). Menopausal status as a factor in the distribution of estrogen and progestin receptors in breast cancer. Surgical Forum 32: 410-412.

Boyle DM, Wiehle RD, Shahabi NA, Wittliff JL (1985). Rapid, high-resolution procedure for assessment of estrogen receptor heterogeneity in clinical samples. J Chromatogr 327: 369-376.

Carlson JA, Allegra JC, Day TG Jr., Wittliff JL (1984). Tamoxifen and endometrial carcinoma alterations in estrogen and progeserone receptors in untreated patients and combination hormonal therapy in advanced neoplasia. Amer J Obstet Gynecol 149:149-153.

Clark GM, McGuire WL, Hubay CA, Pearson OH, Marshall JS (1983). Progesterone receptors as a prognostic factor in stage II breast cancer. N Eng J Med 309: 1343-1347.

Creasman WT, McCarty KS Sr, Barton TK, and McCarty KS Jr, (1980). Clinical correlates of estrogen- and progesterone-binding proteins in human endometrial adenocarcinoma, Obstet. Gynecol 55: 363-370.

Creasman WT, Soper JT, McCarty KS Jr, McCarty KS Sr, Hinshaw W and Clarke-Pearson DL (1985) Influence of cytoplasmic steroid receptor content on prognosis of early stage endometrial carcinoma. Am J Obstet Gynecol 151: 922-932.

Ehrlich CE, Young PC, and Cleary RE (1981) Cytoplasmic progesterone and estradiol receptors in normal, hyperplastic, and carcinomatous endometria: Therapeutic implications. Am J Obstet Gynecol 141: 539-.

Fisher B, Redmond C, Brown A, Wickerham DL, Wolmark N, Allegra JC, Escher G, Lippman M, Savlov E, Wittliff JL, Fisher ER, et al (1983). Influence of tumor estrogen and progesterone receptor levels on the response to tamoxifen and chemotherapy in primary breast cancer. J Clin Oncol 1: 227-241.

Fuchs A, Day TC Jr., Allegra JC, and Wittliff JL (1987). Reference ranges and distribution of steroid hormone receptors in endometrial carcinoma, Submitted.

Greene GL, Fitche FW, Jensen EV (1980). Monoclonal antibodies to estrophiliin: Probes for the study of estrogen receptors. Proc Natl Acad Sci USA 77: 157-161.

Grill H, Manz B, Belozsky O and Pollow K (1984). Criteria for establishment of the double labeling assay for simultaneous determination of estrogen and progesterone receptors. Oncology 41: 25-32.

Hockberg RB, (1979). Iodine-124-labeled estradiol: A gamma-emitting analog of estradiol that binds to the estrogen receptor. Science 205: 1138-1140.

Horwitz KG, McGuire WL, Pearson OH, Segaloff A (1975) predicting response to endocrine therapy in human breast cancer: A hypothesis. Science 189: 726-727.

Jordan VC (1985). Antiestrogens as Antitumor Agents In: Hollander VP (ed), Hormonally Responsive Tumors, Acdemic Press, New York, pp 219-235.

Kauppila A, Kujansuu E, and Vihko R (1982). Cytosol estrogen and progestin receptors in endometrial carcinoma of patients treated with surgery, radiotherapy, and progestin, Cancer 50: 2157-2162.

King WJ and Greene GL (1984). Monoclonal antibodies localized oestrogen receptor in the nuclei of target cells. Nature 307: 745-747.

King WJ, DeSombre ER, Jensen EV (1985). Comparison of immunocytochemical and steroid-binding assays for estrogen receptor in human breast tumors. Cancer Res 45: 293-304.

Lippman M, Bolan G, Huff AA (1976). The effects of estrogens and antiestrogens hormone-responsive human breast cancer in long-term tissue culture. Cancer Res 36: 4595-4691.

Lippman ME, Cassidy J, Eesley M et al., (1984). A randomized attempt to increase the efficacy of cytotoxic chemotherapy in metastatic breast cancer by hormonal synchronization. J Clin Onc 2: 28-36.

Martin JD, Hahnel R, McCartney AJ and Woodings TL (1983). The effect of estrogen receptor status on survival in patients with endometrial cancer. Am J Obstet Gynecol 147: 322-324.

McCarty KS Jr., Miller LS, Cox EB et al. (1985). Estrogen receptor analyses: Correlation of biochemical and immunohistochemical methods using monoclonal antireceptor antibodies, Arch Pathol Lab Med 109: 716-721.

McGuire WL, Carbone PO, Vollmer EP, (eds) (1975) Estrogen receptors in human breast cancer, New York: Raven Press.

Mirecki DM and Jordan VC (1985). Steroid hormone receptors and human breast cancer. Laboratory Medicine 16(5): 287-294.

Mortel R, Levy C, Wolff J-P, Nicholas J-C, Robel P and Baulieu EE (1981). Female sex steroid receptors in postmenopausal endometrial carcinoma and biochemical response to an antiestrogen, Cancer Res 41: 1140-1147.

Raam S and Vrabel DM (1986). Evaluation of an enzyme immunoassay kit for estrogen recedptor measurements. Clin Chem 32: 1496-1502.

Sarfaty GA, Nash AR and Keightly DD (eds) (1981) Estrogen receptor assays in breast cancer: Laboratory discrepencies and quality assurance, New York: Masson Publishing USA, Inc.

Sato N, Hyder SM, Chang L, Thais A, Wittliff JL (1986). Interaction of estrogen receptor isoiforms with immobilized monoclonal antibodies. J Chromatogr 359: 475-487.

Senler TI, Dean WL, Pierce WM and Wittliff JL (1985a). Procedures for measuring cytochrome P-450 dependent hydroxylation activity in reproductive tissues. Anal Biochem 144:152-158.

Senler TI, Dean WL, Murray LF, Wittliff JL (1985b). Quantification of cytochrome P-450-dependent cyclohexane hydroxylase activity in normal and neoplastic reproductive tissues. Biochem J 227: 379-387.

Swenerton KD, Shaw D et al. (1979). Treatment of advanced endometrial carcinoma with tamoxifen. N Eng J Med 301: 105.

van der Walt LA, Sanfilippo JS, Siegel JE and Wittliff JL (1986). Estrogen and progestin receptors in human uterus: Reference ranges of clinical conditions. Clin Physiol Biochem 4: 217-228.

Welshons WV, Lieberman ME, Gorski J (1984). Nuclear localization of unoccupied oestrogen receptors. Nature 307: 747-749.

Wittliff JL (1984). Steroid hormone receptors in breast cancer. Cancer 53: 630-643.

Wittliff, JL (1986). HPLC steroid-hormone receptors. LC-GC Magazine of Liquid and Gas Chromatography, J Steroid Biochem, Aster Publishing Co, Springfield, Oregon, 4(11): 1092-1106.

Wittliff JL (1987a). Steroid hormone receptors. In: Pesce AJ and Kaplan LA (eds). Methods in Clinical Chemistry, CV Mosby Co. St. Louis, pp 767-795.

Wittliff JL (1987b) Steroid Receptor Analyses, Quality control and clinical significance. In: Donegan WL and Spratt JS Jr (eds), Cancer of the Breast, W.B. Saunders Co., Philadelphia, PA, In Press.

Wittliff JL, Durant JR, Fisher B (1981). Methods of steroid receptor analyses and their quality control in the clinical laboratory. In: Soto R, DeNicola AF, Blaquier JA (eds) Physiopathology of Endocrine Diseases and Mechanisms of Hormone Action: New York: Alan R. Liss, pp. 397-411.

Wittliff JL, Lewko WM, Park DC, Kute TE, Baker DT Jr., and Kane LN (1978). Steroid-binding proteins of mammary tissues and their clinical significance in breast cancer, In: W. L. McGuire (ed.), Hormones, Receptors, and Breast Cancer, pp. 325-359, New York: Raven Press.

Wittliff JL, Wiehle RD (1985) Analytical methods of steroid hormone receptors and their quality assurance. In: Hollander VP (ed), Hormonally Responsive Tumors, Academic Press Inc, New York, 15: 383.

Prediction of Response to Cancer Therapy, pages 43–59
© 1988 Alan R. Liss, Inc.

GLUCOCORTICOID-INDUCED LYSIS OF HUMAN LEUKEMIA CELLS

Uri Galili

MacMillan-Cargill Hematology Research Laboratory, Cancer Research Institute, The University of California, San Francisco, California.

Glucocorticoids (GC) play a major role in the chemotherapeutic regimen of acute lymphoblastic leukemias (ALL). Administration of these hormones was found to result in a decrease in the malignant lymphoid cell population in ALL patients (Goldin et al., 1962). Differences in the responsiveness of various leukemias to treatment with GC became evident soon after the introduction of this type of chemotherapy (Claesson and Ropke, 1969). Given the role of cytoplasmic receptors in mediating steroid hormone biologic effects, it was assumed that a plausible explanation for unresponsiveness to GC treatment includes a reduction in the number of receptors and defects in receptor structure. Whereas such factors were found to determine GC resistance of lymphoma cells in a murine experimental model (Harris and Baxter, 1979; Sibley and Yamamoto, 1979), no significant variations in the number or structure of GC receptors have been found in human leukemia cells from responsive and nonresponsive patients (Homo-Delarche, 1984; Sherman et al., 1984; Quddus et al., 1985). Thus it has been concluded that, unlike breast cancer patients, where determining the level of estrogen receptors provides important information for the treatment regimen, quantitation and characterization of GC receptors has a very limited predictive value in GC treatment of individual leukemic patients. In our attempts to establish a predictive analysis of the effect of GC on leukemic cells, we have been studying the actual direct cytolysis induced by GC in malignant cells of leukemic patients. This was studied by incubating leukemic cells with GC and assessing the cytolytic effect by viable cell staining. The sensitvity of the leukemic cells to GC was determined by the proportion of cells killed by these drugs (Galili et al., 1980). The sensitivity of the leukemic cells was correlated with that of normal lymphoid cells of corresponding differentiation stages, and with the in vivo lympholytic effect of GC hormones.

Materials and Methods

Patients studied

Blood samples were obtained from 24 patients with chronic lymphocytic leukemia (CLL), 39 patients with acute lymphoblastic leukemia (ALL), 17 patients with chronic myeloid leukemia (CML) in blast crisis, and 19 patients with acute myeloblastic leukemia. All leukemic patients had white cell blood counts higher than 15,000/mm³ with >80% neoplastic cells. The *in vivo* lympholytic effect of GC in the leukemic patients was determined by the white cell count after short-term (24 h) exposure to the drug in the course of the routine chemotherapeutic regimens used for these patients. Blood was obtained from 50 healthy individuals and from 5 patients with rheumatoid arthritis. Synovial fluid of these rheumatoid arthritis patients was analyzed as well. Normal lymph nodes were obtained from specimens studied for lymphoma staging and found histologically to be free of disease. Thymic tissues were obtained from individuals undergoing open heart surgery. Fetal thymic tissues were obtained from aborted fetuses (17-23 weeks of gestation) in the course of routine pathological examinations.

Cell suspensions

Peripheral blood lymphocytes (PBL) and leukemia cells isolated from heparinized blood were collected from the top of a 9% Ficoll-Hypaque (F/H) barrier (Pharmacia, Sweden). Synovial lymphocytes were separated by a similar method from the washed synovial leukocyte mixture. The monocytes were removed by attachment to a plastic surface during 30 min incubation at 37°C. The polymorphonuclear cells were recovered from the bottom of the F/H barrier. Thymic and lymph node lymphocytes were obtained by passing the minced tissues through stainless-steel mesh. Dead cells were removed by centrifugation on F/H gradient. All cell suspensions were washed twice and brought to a concentration of 2 x 10⁶ cells/ml in RPMI 1640 medium supplemented with 10% fetal calf serum.

Isolation of prothymocytes

Fetal thymic cell suspensions were allowed to form E rosettes with sheep erythrocytes and centrifuged on top of a F/H barrier. The cells that failed to form E rosettes (prothymocytes) remained on top of the F/H barrier. Ninety-eight per cent of the F/H sedimented cells were in rosette form (thymocytes). Rosetting sheep erythrocytes were lysed with 0.85% ammonium chloride. Prothymocytes proved to be the progenitor cell of the thymocytes, since these cells differentiated spontaneously into small

E rosetting thymocytes during 5 days' incubation *in vitro* (Galili *et al.*, 1980a).

In vitro *lymphocyte activation in one-way mixed lymphocyte culture (MLC)*

Normal PBL (10^6 cells/ml in RPMI 1640 medium supplemented with 10% heat-inactivated AB serum) were mixed with equal amounts of X-ray-irradiated (3500 rads) PBL from a second individual. The cell mixture was incubated for 5 days in 5% CO_2 humidified atmosphere at 37°C. During this period, the T lymphocytes undergo activation against the allohistocompatibility antigens on the surface of the irradiated PBL.

In vitro *GC-induced cytolysis*

Aliquots of 0.2 ml lymphoid or myeloid cells (2×10^6 cells/ml) were incubated with various concentrations of cortisol (Ikapharm, Israel), in flat-bottom microwells (Cooke Engineering Co., Alexandria, VA) for 20 h, or as indicated, at 37°C in 5% CO_2 humidified atmosphere. The proportion of lysed cells was assessed by determining the concentration of the remaining viable cells in a hemocytometer using the Trypan Blue exclusion test. The percentage of cytolysis was calculated by means of the formula

$$[(a - b)/a] \times 100$$

where a is the concentration of viable cells in control wells containing medium without cortisol and b is the concentration of viable cells in wells containing the hormone. The effect of other steroids was similarly studied.

Metabolic inhibitors

Actinomycin D (0.01 μg/ml), an inhibitor of RNA synthesis, puromycin and cycloheximide (0.1 μg/ml), both inhibitors of protein synthesis (all from Sigma Chemical Co., St. Louis, MO) were used to determine the involvement of transcriptional and translational events in the course of GC-induced cytolysis.

Phenotyping of the ALL cells

The ALL cells were phenotyped using a variety of monoclonal antibodies for the common ALL antigen (CALLA), Ia antigen, and T cell antigen (Foon and Todd, 1986). In addition, cells were examined for cytoplasmic IgM (cyt. IgM) and for the capacity to form E rosettes (E ros). All the ALL cells were positively stained with antibodies to terminal deoxynucleotidyl transferase. The ALL cells were divided into the following subclasses (Table I).

Table I

ALL Type	Surface Markers
Common ALL (cALL)	T$^-$ Ia$^+$ CALLA$^+$ Cyt.IgM$^-$ E-ros$^-$
Pre B ALL	T$^-$ Ia$^+$ CALLA$^\pm$ Cyt.IgM$^+$ E-ros$^-$
Pre T ALL (early T ALL)	T$^+$ Ia$^-$ CALLA$^-$ Cyt.IgM$^-$ E-ros$^-$
T ALL	T$^+$ Ia$^-$ CALLA$^-$ Cyt.IgM$^-$ E-ros$^+$

Results and Discussion

GC-induced lysis of human normal lymphocytes

Most of the current knowledge on GC-induced lysis of lymphoid cells has been obtained from experimental animal models such as rat and mouse thymocytes and lymphoma cells. Man has been regarded as a "GC-resistant species" (Claman, 1972), since human thymocytes and PBL were found to be resistant to lysis by GC. Nevertheless, we have found distinct differentiation stages in which human T cells are highly sensitive to GC lysis *in vitro,* and this sensitivity may explain some *in vitro* phenomena observed upon administration of these drugs.

The earliest T cell differentiation stage in which the human lymphoid cells are highly sensitive to GC lysis is the prothymocyte (Galili *et al.,* 1980a). The prothymocyte is the precursor cell which migrates from the bone marrow into the thymus, where it proliferates and differentiates into cortical thymocytes. The prothymocytes are large cells (>8 μm) containing loose nuclear chromatin and a basophilic cytoplasm (Fig. 1). Thymocytes, in contrast, are small cells (5-6.5 μm) with dense nuclear chromatin and almost no detectable cytoplasm.

The prothymocytes comprise a small proportion of the post-natal thymus. However, large proportions of prothymocytes could be isolated from fetal thymuses (Galili *et al.,* 1980a). Prothymocytes were isolated from fetal thymic suspensions on the basis of their inability to form E rosettes with sheep erythrocytes, a characteristic expressed by human thymocytes and mature T cells. When analyzed for sensitivity, the lysis by 10^{-5} M cortisol, prothymocytes were readily killed after 20 h incubation with the hormone, whereas the viability of cortical thymocytes was not affected (Table II).

The mature circulating lymphocytes found in the blood or lymphoid organs, like blood monocytes and granulocytes, were found to be completely resistant to GC-induced lysis. Once the T lymphocytes are activated, they become sensitive to GC lysis. This sensitivity can be demonstrated in *in vitro* activated lymphocytes in mixed lymphocyte cultures, or with T cells isolated from *in vivo* immunoreactive sites such as

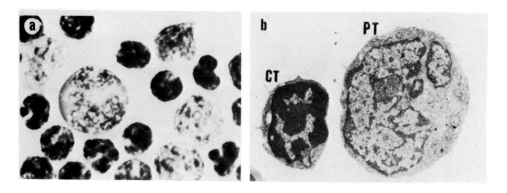

Fig. 1: a. A suspension of human fetal thymic cells. Large cells are the prothymocytes; small cells are cortical thymocytes (x1000). b. An electron micrograph of a prothymocyte (PT) and a cortical thymocyte (x3600). (From Galili *et al.*, 1980a)

Table II

Sensitivity of Various Human Normal Lymphoid and Myeloid Cells to GC-induced Lysis

Cell Type	% Cell Lysis[a]
Prothymocytes	78 ± 4.3
Thymocytes	0
PBL	0
Lymph node lymphocytes	0
Synovial fluid lymphocytes	75 ± 2.2
Activated T cells in MLC	83 ± 5.8
Activated B cells (EBV-transformed)	0
Blood monocytes	0
Blood granulocytes	0
Normal bone marrow cells	0

[a] Cells were incubated for 20 h with 10^{-5}M cortisol, then assayed for viability. Results are the mean $\pm$ SG of 3-10 different experiments.

the synovial fluid of arthritic patients (Galili *et al.*, 1980b). A similar GC sensitivity of *in vivo* activated T cells has been detected among T lymphocytes infiltrating solid tumor (Galili *et al.*, 1980c), T lymphocytes in the blood of infectious mononucleosis of patients in an active state of the disease (Galili *et al.*, 1980d), and within the involved lymphoid organs of Hodgkin's lymphoma patients (Galili *et al.*, 1980e). These findings clearly indicate that, in contrast to the view of man being a GC-resistant species, there are distinct lymphoid subpopulaions within the T cell differentiation pathway which are highly sensitive to GC-induced lysis. Activated B cells, which produce immunoglobulins and proliferate as a result of transformation by Epstein-Barr virus, are resistant to lysis (Table II). Moreover, the immunoglobulin secretion from these B cells is not affected by the GC hormone (not shown), suggesting that the observed decrease in serum immunoglobulins in GC-treated patients may result from specific lysis of B lymphocytes at a rather early stage of differentiation.

GC-induced lysis of leukemic cells

Malignant cells from various leukemic patients were assayed for sensitivity to GC lysis by incubation with 10^{-5}M cortisol for 20 h at 37°C. CLL cells from all patients were found to be highly sensitive, as indicated by the large proportion of lysed cells (Fig. 2). A similar high sensitivity was found in malignant cells isolated from half of the patients with acute lymphoblastic leukemia. However, ALL cells from the remaining patients were resistant to GC-induced lysis (Fig. 2). Cells from patients with acute or chronic myeloid leukemias remained unaffected. The observed GC resistance of the AML and CML cells is in accord with the well-documented refractory response of myeloid leukemia patients to GC treatment.

It was of interest to determine within the ALL patient group whether the GC sensitivity observed in half of the patients correlates with various leukemic subsets. The leukemic cells from 20 patients with common ALL were found to be resistant following incubation with 10^{-5}M cortisol (Fig. 3). In contrast, the cells from ten pre-B leukemias were readily lysed by cortisol. Cells from six patients with pre-T leukemia were similarly sensitive to cortisol-induced lysis, whereas cells from three patients with the more mature T-cell phenotype in the T-leukemia were found to be resistant. These findings suggest that GC sensitivity of leukemic cells parallels that of their normal counterpart according to their differentiation state. Pre-T leukemic cells, also called early-T leukemias (Foon and Todd, 1986) which have phenotypic features similar to prothymocytes, are highly sensitive to GC lysis; whereas T leukemias with phenotypic markers similar to the cortical thymocytes are completely resistant. The sensitivity of pre-B ALL or CLL, both of which are early stages in B cell differentiation, versus the resistance of the cALL cells may likewise be attributed to a differentiation state-related phenomenon.

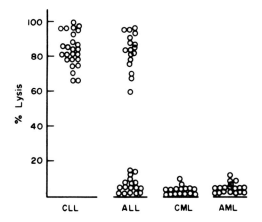

Fig. 2. Cortisol (10^{-5}M)-induced cytolysis of various leukemic cells. Each circle represents the results obtained from one patient (From Galili *et al.*, 1980.)

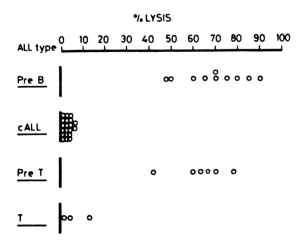

Fig. 3. Cortisol-induced lysis of leukemic cells of various ALL types.

GC sensitivity in in vitro *proliferating human leukemia cell lines*

The main objective in chemotherapy treatment is the eradication of the proliferating compartment of the leukemic cells, which is usually in the bone marrow or within the lymphoid organs. The sensitivity of proliferating malignant cells may differ from that of the circulating cells, which are mostly at G_0 stage of the cell cycle. Thus it was of interest to determine GC cytolytic effect on human cell lines of different lymphoid subsets. Four different cell lines were studied for their sensitivity to GC-induced lysis. The B lymphoid cell line Daudi (Klein *et al.*, 1968), the T lymphoid cell line HD-MAR (Ben-Bassat *et al.*, 1980), and the myeloid cell line K562 (Lozzio and Lozzio, 1975), were not affected by GC. When grown in the presence of GC (10^{-6}M dexamethasone), their proliferation rate did not differ from control cultures which were grown in the absence of GC (Fig. 4). However most of the cells of the pre-T leukemia cell line Be-13 were killed within 24 h (Galili *et al.*, 1984) (Fig. 4). This supports the previous observation on the relationship between GC sensitivity and the differentiation state of the malignant lymphoid cell.

The lytic mechanism within GC-sensitive cells

The general biological effect of steroid hormones is mediated by cytoplasmic receptors for the steroid molecule. The steroid molecule rapidly penetrates through the cell membrane and interacts with specific cytoplasmic receptors. Thereafter the steroid receptor complex penetrates into the nucleus, binds to the chromatin, and activates certain genes. The subsequent gene product(s) synthesized constitute the biologic response of various tissues to the steroid hormone (Edelman, 1975). Studies on the mechanism of GC-induced lysis of rodent thymocytes or lymphoma cells have indicated that the lysis of cells by GC occurs according to this mechanism (Harris and Baxter, 1979; Sibley and Yamamoto, 1979). The GC lysis of human leukemia cells was also found to be mediated by specific receptors and to involve specific gene activation. This could be demonstrated by the fact that incubation of GC-sensitive cells such as CLL or activated T cells for 15-30 min with 10^{-5}M cortisol was found sufficient to induce an irreversible lytic process (Galili *et al.*, 1982; Galili, 1983). The specific interaction of GC with the cytoplasmic receptor could be further demonstrated by the use of the antagonist cortexolone, which binds to the cytoplasmic receptor but does not elicit a biologic effect (Turnell *et al.*, 1979). GC-sensitive cells were incubated with cortisol alone or together with a tenfold concentration of cortexolone for 30 min at 37°C. Thereafter the cells were washed and the lytic effect was scored after 20 h incubation at 37°C. As seen in Table III, cortexolone inhibited the lysis by competitive inhibition of cortisol binding to the receptor. This experiment could be performed only at a 30-minute pulse with the steroids, since

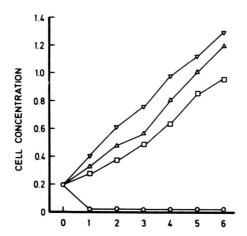

Fig. 4. *In vitro* growth of various human cell lines in the presence of 10⁻⁶M dexamethasone. O, Be 13 cells; □, HD-Mar cells; Δ, Daudi cells; ∇, K562 cells. Number of viable cells/ml in all cell lines except Be 13 did not differ in control cultures from that observed in cultures containing the hormone. Growth curve of Be 13 control cultures is the same as that of Daudi cells (From Galili *et al.*, 1984.)

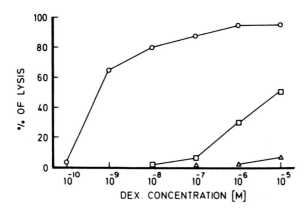

Fig. 5. Inhibitory effect of actinomycin (0.1 µg/ml)(□) and cyclo-heximide (1 µg/ml)(Δ) on dexamethasone-inducd lysis of B3 13 cells. O, cultures containing dexamethasone without metabolic inhibitors (From Galili *et al.*, 1984).

Table III

Inhibition of Cortisol-induced Lysis by Cortexolone

Drug Content

Cell Type	cortisol (10^{-5}M)	cortexolone (10^{-4}M)	cortisol (10^{-5}M) cortexolone (10^{-4}M)
Activated T cells	59 ± 2.9[a]	16 ± 4.2	22 ± 6.1
CLL cells	57 ± 2.4	8.3 ± 3.5	10 ± 3.9

[a] Mean $\pm$ SE of five different experiments.

10^{-4}M cortexolone exerts a nonspecific lysis of cells when incubated for prolonged periods with various cells.

Based on studies with GC-resistant mutants of mouse lymphoma cells (Harris and Baxter, 1979; Sibley and Yamamoto, 1979), it has been argued that GC resistance of human leukemic cells may result from low numbers of receptors per cell (Lippman et al., 1973). No significant difference in number of receptors was found in the Be 13 GC-sensitive cell line and the K562 Daudi or HD-Mar GC-resistant cells (Galili et al., 1984). Furthermore, activated T cells which are GC-sensitive have a similar number of receptors as resting PBL (Galili et al., 1980b). In addition, nuclear translocation of the GC/receptor complex was observed in both GC-sensitive and -resistant cells (Galili et al., 1984). Thus in accord with studies of other groups, human leukemias do not differ in the number of cytoplasmic receptors to an extent which may explain the difference in GC sensitivity. Studies on the structure of cytoplasmic receptors did not detect defects in the receptors' structure, which may explain unresponsiveness of some types of leukemia to steroid therapy (Sherman et al., 1984). Thus the major difference between human GC-sensitive and -resistant lymphoid cells seems to lie in the differentiation state of the cells.

The lytic process of human GC-sensitive cells seems to involve the activation of a gene(s) which encodes for a protein that causes an autolytic effect on the cell. This could be demonstrated indirectly by inhibition of cell lysis as a result of the administration of the RNA synthesis inhibitor actinomycin-D, and protein synthesis inhibitors puromycine and cycloheximide (Galili et al., 1982; Galili, 1983).

An example of the effect of transcription and translation inhibitors on GC-induced lysis is shown in Figure 5. The pre-T leukemia cell line

Be 13 is highly sensitive to lysis by the synthetic GC, dexamethasone, which causes cell lysis even at a concentration of $10^{-9}M$. When the RNA synthesis inhibitor actinoymycin-D was added, complete inhibition of lysis induced by $10^{-7}M$ and $10^{-8}M$ dexamethasone was observed. A partial inhibition of lysis occurred with $10^{-5}M$ and $10^{-6}M$ of the hormone. The protein synthesis inhibitor cycloheximide exhibited a more potent inhibitory effect and abolished the lysis induced by dexamethasone, even at the high concentration of $10^{-5}M$. The nature of the "autolytic" protein which causes the cell death as a result of exposure to GC is not clear as yet, since it has not yet been isolated or identified. However, the antagonistic effect of transcription and translation inhibitors raises the need for a critical evaluation of the clinical benefit of the administration of drugs with such an activity concurrently with GC, in the course of chemotherapeutic regimens.

Kinetics of the lytic process

The process of lysis in freshly isolated CLL and ALL cells can be detected by means of the vital staining technique only after 6 h of incubation with the hormone at 37°C (Galili *et al.*, 1980, 1982). However, ultrastructural alterations within the affected cells can already be demonstrated within the first 2 h of incubation. Figure 6 describes sequential morphological changes in CLL cells incubated with $2 \times 10^{-5}M$ cortisol at 37°C for varying time periods. After 2 h, the affected cell loses its microvillous structure of the membrane, and after 4 h, small pores are observed in the membrane. Water penetrating through these holes leads to the eventual death of the cell, which can be clearly demonstrated within 6 h of incubation. By transmission electron microscopy, the first morphological changes detected within the cytoplasm seem to be swelling of the mitcochondria, and would suggest early damage of the respiratory compartment of the cell. No morphological changes were detected within the nucleus at this stage, which may reflect the DNA fragmentation, suggested by others to occur at early stages of GC-induced lysis (Ucker, 1987).

The proliferating GC-sensitive Be 13 cells display a different kinetic pattern of cytolysis. Lysis could not be observed in the light microscope before 16 h incubation (Galili *et al.*, 1984). At 20 h incubation, 60% to 80% of the cells were killed, and only after 24 h, lysis of the entire population was observed. The presence of the GC hormone in the medium for the entire incubation period was essential for obtaining complete lysis. Removal of dexamethasone after 8 h resulted in no lysis of the Be 13 cells. This is in contrast to the observations with freshly isolated CLL and ALL cells where 30 min incubation with GC hormones was sufficient to irreversibly induce cell lysis (Galili, 1983). These findings suggest that the lytic process is induced during a specific stage(s) of the cell cycle. A substantial proportion of the cells must pass this specific stage before a measurable lytic effect is seen. It should be noted that during the 24 h

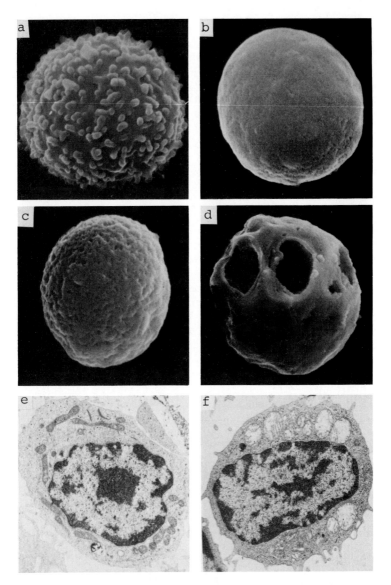

Fig. 6. Morphologic aspects of GC-induced lysis of CLL cells. Cells were incubated for various periods with 10⁻⁵M cortisol and processed for scanning or transmission electron microscopy (x7000-8000). a. control cell. b. 2 hr incubation with cortisol. c. 4 hr. d. 6 hr. e. control cell. f. 2 hr. (Modified from Galili *et al.*, 1982)

incubation with GC, no arrest in cell cycle of Be 13 cells was observed. Thus the proportion of mitotic figures and ^{3}H thymidine incorporation per 10^6 live cells did not differ in Be 13 cultures incubated for 16 h with dexamethasone and in control cultures in the absence of hormone (Galili *et al.*, 1984). These findings suggest that the lytic process affects metabolic pathways different from those controlling the cell cycle. Studies on another human T cell line, CEM-7, performed by Harmon *et al.* (1979) have shown a different effect of dexamethasone, also resulting in cell death. As a result of exposure to GC, the CEM-7 ceases to proliferate and is arrested in the G_1 phase of the cell cycle. The cell dies only after 4 to 5 days' incubation with the drug. Thus CEM-7 cells are probably killed by a mechanism different from that observed in the Be 13 cells, which are lysed within 20 h incubation and are not arrested in their cell cycle. Nevertheless, both studies indicate that proliferating leukemic cells must be exposed to GC for relatively prolonged periods in order to elicit an efficient lytic response.

Correlation between in vitro *and* in vivo *cytolytic effect of GC on leukemia cells*

The ultimate correlation between the *in vitro* cytolytic effect of GC and *in vivo* lysis of leukemic cells requires the demonstration of a decrease in the malignant cell count in the blood, in cases where *in vitro* GC sensitivity is observed. *In vivo*, there are many unrelated factors which may affect malignant cell count, and which may obscure the data. Examples of such factors are the effects of GC on the redistribution of white blood cells in the marginal pool and the circulation (Claman, 1972), and the hydration required in the treatment of leukemia patients, which may increase blood volume and thus decrease cell count.

Attempts to study the *in vivo* GC cytolytic effect were carried out in two CLL and six ALL patients by determining the cell count 24 h after administration of GC to the patients (70 mg/m² prednisone). As can be seen in Table IV, there was a good correlation between the *in vitro* and *in vivo* effect in the two CLL patients and four of the ALL patients. However, two ALL patients (Nos. 7 and 8) showed decreases in the cell count without apparent *in vitro* lysis.

A further support for the correlation between the *in vitro* and *in vivo* GC cytolytic effect was observed in patient No. 1. This CLL patient, who exhibited a marked decrease in WBC count after GC treatment, returned after two months for further treatment as a result of elevation of his WBC count. The CLL cells at this stage showed moderate sensitivity to GC lysis, both *in vitro* and *in vivo*. When this patient was admitted for the third treatment 6 weeks later, his CLL cells displayed complete resistance to GC-induced lysis *in vitro* as well as *in vivo*. Thus the possible selection of GC-resistant malignant clones, in the course of treatment, was reflected in the *in vitro* alteration in the sensitivity of the CLL cells.

Table IV

Correlation Between the *In Vitro* and *In Vivo* Cytolytic Effect of GC
on Leukemic Cells

| Leukemia Type | Pt. no. | WBC Count | | In Vitro[a] Lysis (%) |
		Before GC Administration	24 h After GC Administration	
CLL	1	70,000	11,000	92
	1A	80,000	35,000	60
	1B	75,000	70,000	5
	2	55,000	14,000	85
ALL	3	32,000	9,000	65
	4	21,000	5,500	73
	5	25,000	18,000	10
	6	18,000	8,000	48
	7	22,000	13,000	5
	8	15,000	9,000	8

[a] The *in vitro* GC lysis was studied by incubation of the cells with 10^{-5}M cortisol. 1A and 1B represent sequential GC treatments of patient No. 1.

Conclusions

1.   In contrast to the general notion that man is a "GC-resistant species," our studies demonstrate specific human lymphoid subsets which are readily lysed by upper physiologic and pharmacologic concentrations of GC. In the T lymphoid lineage, these include prothymocytes and activated T lymphocytes. It is speculated that pre-B cells may be the GC-sensitive differentiation stage within the B lymphoid lineage. The GC sensitivity may reflect a physiologic regulatory mechanism, through which the extent of immune response is controlled. It is possible that "overshooting" of the immune response would cause stress resulting in the elevation of endogenous GC. This in turn would affect the GC-sensitive lymphoid subsets, and thus limit the immune response. The *in vivo* physiologic effect of endogenous GC on prothymocytes has been demonstrated in an experimental animal model (Cano Castellanos *et al.*, 1983).

2.   The GC sensitivity or resistance of lymphoid subsets is preserved in the malignant counterparts of corresponding differentiation stages. Like

prothymocytes, pre-T leukemias are sensitive to GC-induced lysis; whereas T leukemia cells like thymocytes are resistant. Pre-B leukemias and CLL cells, which represent a differentiation stage preceding that of B cells, are also GC-sensitive. Malignant B lymphocytes such as Burkitt's lymphoma cells, and EBV-transformed B cells like mature B cells are GC-resistant. Myeloid leukemia cells, like normal myeloid cells, are also GC-resistant. Common ALL cells, which are considered to be very early stages of B cell differentiation (Foon and Todd, 1986) are GC-resistant.

3.   GC-induced lysis of human leukemia cells is mediated via the binding of the GC molecule to a cytoplasmic receptor, translocation of the GC/receptor complex into the nucleus, and activation of specific gene(s) which encode for an "autolytic protein." This "autolytic protein" is still hypothetical, since it has not yet been identified and isolated. In freshly isolated leukemic cells, the generation of this protein and the initiation of the cellular damage which leads to cell death occurs within 2 h of exposure to the hormone. Metabolic inhibitors of RNA and protein synthesis inhibit the GC-induced lysis.

4.   There is no significant difference in receptor number in GC-sensitive and -resistant cells. It is possible that the detection of GC sensitivity only in distinct normal and malignant differentiation stages reflects the accessibility of the relevant genes for activation by the GC/receptor complex. In proliferating GC-sensitive leukemia cells, this gene(s) seems to be accessible to activation only within a specific phase of the cell cycle. Thus proliferating leukemia cells have to be exposed for prolonged periods to the GC hormone in order to achieve effective lysis.

5.   Few correlations between the *in vitro* cytolytic effect of GC on leukemic cells and *in vivo* lysis of cells suggest that cells which display *in vitro* sensitivity to GC are also lysed *in vivo*. These studies are limited to the immediate and direct lytic effec of GC hormones. A longer-term inhibitory effect on leukemia cell proliferation in leukemias defined as GC-resistant is not excluded. However GC do not inhibit *in vitro* proliferation of GC-resistant cell lines. Careful analysis of the mitotic activity of malignant cells in the bone marrow of leukemic patients treated with GC would help to determine whether, apart from the cytolytic effect, these hormones also cause inhibition of malignant cell proliferation in leukemias which are resistant to the *in vitro* GC lysis.

References

Ben-Bassat H, Mitrani-Rosenbaum S, Gamliel H, Naparstek E, Leizerowitz R, Kurkesh A, Sagi M, Voss R, Kohn G, Polliack A (1980). Establishment in continuous culture of a T-lymphoid cell line (HD-Mar) from a patient with Hodgkin's lymphoma. Int J Cancer 25: 583.

Cano Castellanos R, Leizerowitz R, Kaiser N, Galili N, Polliack A, Korkesh A, Galili U (1983). Prothymocytes in postirradiation regenerating rat thymuses: A model for studying early stages in T cell differentiation. J Immunol 130:121.

Claesson MH, Ropke C (1969). Quantitative studies on cortisol-induced decay of lymphoid cells in the thymolymphatic system. Acta Pathol Microbiol Scand 76:376.

Claman HN (1972). Corticosteroids and lymphoid cells. N Engl J Med 287:388.

Edelman IS (1975). Mechanism of action of steroid hormones. J Steroid Biochem 6:147.

Foon KA, Todd RF III (1986). Immunologic classification of leukemias and lymphomas. Blood 68:1.

Galili U, Prokocimer M, Izak G (1980). The in vitro sensitivity of leukemic and normal leukocytes to hydrocortisone-induced cytolysis. Blood 56:1077.

Galili U, Polliack A, Okon E, Leizerowitz R, Gamliel H, Korkesh A, Schenker JG, Izak G (1980a). Human prothymocytes: membrane properties, differentiation patterns, glucocorticoid sensitivity and ultrastructural features. J Exp Med 152:796.

Galili N, Galili U, Klein E, Rosenthal L, Nordenskjold B (1980b). Human T lymphocytes become glucocorticoid-sensitive upon immune activation. Cell Immunol 16:173.

Galili U, Klein E, Klein G, Singh Bal I (1980c). Activated T lymphocytes in infiltrates and draining lymph nodes of nasopharingeal carcinoma. Int J Cancer 25:85.

Galili U, Seeley J, Svedmyr E, Klein E, Klein G, Weiland O (1980d). Blood lymphocytes in infectious mononucleosis share the following characteristics with activated T cells: Natural attachment, stable E rosetting and glucocorticoid sensitivity. J Clin Lab Immunol 3:153.

Galili U, Klein E, Christensson B, Biberfeld P (1980e). Lymphocytes in Hodgkin's biopsies exhibit: stable E rosette formation, natural attachment and glucocorticoid sensitivity, similar to immunoactivated T cells. Clin Immunol Immunopathol 16:173.

Galili U, Leizerowitz R, Moreb J, Gamliel H, Gurfel D, Polliack A (1982). Metabolic and ultrastructural aspects of the in vitro lysis of chronic lymphocytic leukemia cells by glucocorticoids. Cancer Res 42: 1433.

Galili U (1983). Glucocorticoid-induced lysis of human normal and malignant lymphocytes. J Steroid Biochem 19:483.

Galili U, Peleg A, Milner Y, Galili N (1984). Be 13, a human T-leukemia cell line highly sensitive to dexamethasone-induced cytolysis. Cancer Res 44:4594.

Goldin A, Sondberg J, Henderson E, Newman J, Frie E, Holland J (1962). The chemotherapy of human and animal acute leukemia. Cancer Chemother Rep 136:213.

Harmon JM, Norman MR, Fowlkes B, Thompson EB (1979). Dexamethasone induces irreversible G_1 arrest and death of human lymphoid cell line. J Cell Physiol 98:267.

Harris AW, Baxter JD (1979). Variations in cellular sensitivity to glucocorticoids: observations and mechanisms. Monogr Endocrinol 12: 423.

Homo-Delarche F (1984). Glucocorticoid receptors and steroid sensitivity in normal and neoplastic lymphoid tissues: A review. Cancer Res 44: 431.

Klein E, Klein G, Nadkarni JS, Nadkarni JJ, Wigzel H, Clifford P (1968). Surface IgM kappa sensitivity on Burkitt's lymphoma cells *in vivo* and in derived culture lines. Cancer Res 28:1300.

Lippman ME, Halterman RH, Leventhal BG, Perry S, Thompson EB (1973). Glucocorticoid binding proteins in human acute lymphoblastic leukemic blast cells. J Clin Invest 52:1715.

Lozzio CB, Lozzio BB (1975). Human chronic myleogenous leukemia cell line with positive Philadelphia chromosome. Blood 45:321.

Quddus FF, Leventhal BG, Boyett JM, Pullen DJ, Crist WM, Borowitz MJ (1985). Glucocorticoid receptors in immunological subtypes of childhood acute lymphocytic leukemia cells: A pediatric oncology group study. Cancer Res 45:6482.

Sherman MR, Stevens YW, Tuazon FB (1984). Multiple forms and fragments of cytosolic glucocorticoid receptors from human leukemic cells and normal lymphocytes. Cancer Res 44:3783.

Sibley CH, Yamamoto KR (1979). Mouse lymphoma cells: mechanisms of resistance to glucocorticoids. Monogr Endocrinol 12:357.

Turnell RW, Kaiser N, Milholland RJ, Rosen F (1974). Glucocorticoid receptors in rat thymocytes. Interaction with the antiglucocorticoid cortexolone and mechanism of its action. J Biol Chem 249:1133.

Ucker DS (1987). Cytotoxic T lymphocytes and glucocorticoids activate an endogenous suicide process in target cells. Nature 327:62.

Prediction of Response to Cancer Therapy, pages 61-73

P-GLYCOPROTEIN GENE AMPLIFICATION OR OVEREXPRESSION IS NOT DETECTED IN CLINICAL BREAST CANCER SPECIMENS

Douglas E. Merkel, Suzanne A.W. Fuqua, Steven M. Hill, and William L. McGuire

Department of Medicine/Oncology, University of Texas Health Science Center at San Antonio, San Antonio, Texas 78284-7884

More than a decade ago, Ling and colleagues described the induction of cross-resistance to a variety of antitumor antibiotics in a hamster cell line by exposure to increasing concentrations of colchicine (Ling, 1975). This pleotropic, or multiple drug resistance (MDR) was associated with the presence of a 170 kDa membrane glycoprotein (Juliano and Ling, 1976), termed the P-glycoprotein, and decreased intracellular accumulation of antineoplastic agents in resistant cells (Ling and Thompson, 1974). Since these initial observations, the MDR plenotype has been produced in a variety of human cell lines by using similar selection protocols (Beck et al., 1979); Akiyama et al., 1983; Dalton et al., 1986; Twentyman et al., 1986).

Several groups have shown that resistance of MDR cells to cochicine, adriamycin, and other agents can be reversed by exposure to calcium channel-blocking agents, which also reverses the defect in intracellular drug accumulation (Tsuruo et al., 1982; Rogan et al., 1984; Willingham et al., 1986). Binding of the P-glycoprotein to vinblastine, one of the involved antineoplastics, has been demonstrated by photoaffinity labelling (Safa et al., 1986). Such binding is blocked, and antineoplastic sensitivity restored in MDR cells, by monoclonal antibodies directed against the P-glycoprotein (Hamada and Tsuruo, 1986). Further evidence that P-glycoprotein functions as a drug efflux pump is provided by its deduced amino acid sequence and structure (Gros et al., 1986; Chen et al., 1986), which is similar to that of bacterial membrane transport proteins.

The gene coding for P-glycoprotein has been identified by several techniques (Roninson et al., 1986; Riordan et al., 1985;

Scotto et al., 1986). Transfection and expression of this gene is sufficient to produce the MDR phenotype in drug-sensitive cell lines (Gros et al., 1986). The degree of amplification and expression of this gene in cell lines can be correlated with their level of drug resistance (Roninson et al., 1984; Gros et al., 1986). This suggests that amplification or overexpression of this gene might serve as a useful marker for clinical multiple drug resistance, if evidence of the P-glycoprotein/MDR system could be found in naturally occurring human tumors.

P-glycoprotein messenger RNA expression was detected in a number of human tissues by Fojo et al. (Fojo et al., 1987). This group also found overexpression of the P-glycoprotein gene in several human tumor specimens, most notably those arising from tissues which were also P-glycoprotein overexpressors, e.g., adrenal medulla, kidney, and colon. Using monoclonal antibodies, Gerlach et al. detected the P-glycoprotein in some sarcomas and ovarian cancers (Gerlach et al., in press; Bell et al., 1985), but not in three breast cancers.

Resistance to antineoplastic agents, including adriamycin and vinca alkyloids, is frequently encountered in breast cancer. We therefore began a series of studies to determine whether the P-glycoprotein gene was amplified or overexpressed in breast cancer, and thus whether this form of drug resistance could be either predicted or circumvented in breast cancer. Furthermore, we attempted to define the relationship between P-glycoprotein and in vitro drug resistance as determined by clonogenic or thymidine incorporation assays (Von Hoff et al., 1983; Kern et al., 1985). The results of these studies suggest that the P-glycoprotein gene is not responsible for the common occurrence of clinical and in vitro drug resistance in breast cancer.

MATERIALS AND METHODS

Cell Lines

The drug sensitive Chinese hamster ovary cell line CHO-AB and the colchicine resistant subline CHO-C^5 were gifts from Dr. V. Ling, and have been previously described (Lathan et al., 1985). The MDA-231 human breast cancer cell line was obtained from the American Type Culture Collection, Rockville, Maryland. These cells were maintained as monolayer culture in Eagle's minimum essential medium supplemented with 10% fetal bovine serum and 6 ng/ml insulin (Fuqua et al., 1987). The adriamycin-resistant subline MDA-AD^R was generated by stepwise selection in increasing concentrations of adriamycin. This line overexpressed P-glycoprotein mRNA, but this gene was not amplified (Fuqua et al., 1987). Continued passage of MDA-AD^R in adriamycin generated the line MDA-A1 in which the P-glycoprotein gene was both amplified and overexpressed (Merkel et al., 1987). The CHO C5, MDA-AD^R, and MDA-A1 lines were constantly exposed to adriamycin to prevent reversion, as has been reported by others (Gros et al., 1986). All cell lines were routinely tested for, and found to be free of, contamination by Mycoplasma.

P-Glycoprotein cDNA Probes

The hamster P-glycoprotein cDNA clone was isolated from a CHO-C5 mRNA expression library (Young and Davis, 1983) using a previously prepared monoclonal antibody to P-glycoprotein (Lathan et al., 1985). A 1.2 kb Eco RI restriction fragment of the hamster cDNA insert was subcloned into pGEM-4 (Promega-Biotech).

The human cDNA clone was isolated from lambda gt 11 and lambda gt 10 expression libraries prepared from MDA-AD^R cells. The hamster P-glycoprotein cDNA probe was used to select human P-glycoprotein-specific cDNA clones from the lambda libraries. One such clone contained a 1.3 kb insert, which was subcloned into pGEM-4. These hamster and human P-glycoprotein cDNAs were labeled by nich translation (Maniatis et al., 1982) and used as hybridization probes at $1-4 \times 10^6$ cpm/ml.

Human Tumor Specimens

Frozen breast tumor specimens were obtained from the San Antonio Breast Tumor Bank and maintained at -70°C until DNA or RNA isolation was performed. No clinical data were available for the majority of the stage I-II specimens. However, 11 biopsies of metastatic disease which had been obtained withing 3 months following adriamycin treatment were identified.

Twenty-two specimens of locally advanced disease were contributed by Dr. A.U. Buzdar (M.D. Anderson Hospital, Texas). Patients with T_3 or T_4 breast cancer were treated with an induction regimen containing 5-fluorouracil, adriamycin, and cyclophosphamide (Hortobagyi et al., 1983). After achieving a maximal clinical response, mastectomy was performed and a portion of this residual breast cancer was made available.

Other breast tumor specimens were originally sent to the laboratories of Dr. D.D. Von Hoff (San Antonio) and Dr. D.H. Kern (U.C.L.A.) for in vitro sensitivity testing (see below). Specimens which had been assayed for sensitivity to either adriamycin or vinblastine were selected.

DNA Extraction And Southern Hybridization

High molecular weight DNA was extracted (Krieg et al., 1983) from cell lines and tissues and quantitated by diphenylamine assay (Giles and Meyers, 1965). Ten micrograms of DNA was digested with Eco RI restriction endonuclease (Boehringer-Mannheim) under conditions suggested by the manufacturer. Completion of the digestion was confirmed by inspection of the electrophoretic pattern of the DNA in an ethidium bromide-stained agarose minigel. Each DNA digest was then electrophoresed in a 1% agarose gel and transferred onto nitrocellulose (Southern, 1975). The membranes were hybridized with ^{32}P-labelled cDNA probe for 48 hours at $42°C$ in a solution of 45% formamide/0.6 M NaCl/60 mM trisodium citrate (pH 7.0)/0.1 M sodium phosphate (pH 6.5)/0.1% sodium pyrophosphatase/0.1% SDS/1X Denhardt's/100 µg/ml denatured salmon sperm DNA/10% dextran sulfate. The membranes were then washed at room temperature with 0.3 M NaCl/30 mM trisodium citrate/0.1% SDS followed by washes at $60°C$ in 15 mM NaCl/1.5 mM trisodium citrate. Autoradiography was performed at $-70°C$ for 24-72 hours.

Equal loading and transfer of DNA was confirmed by staining of the agarose gel with ethidium bromide both before and after transfer to nitrocellulose. As a further control for any variation in loading and transfer, blots were rehybridized with a rat actin probe (donated by Dr. E. Kraig) and scanned with an absorption densitometer.

RNA Extraction And Northern Hybridization

Total cellular RNA was extracted by homogenization in guanidine isothiocyanate and separated by centrifugation over a cesium chloide gradient (Glisin et al., 1974). RNA was quantitated by absorption spectroscopy at 260 nm, and results confirmed by inspection of an ethidium bromide-stained agarose minigel. When sufficient RNA was available, poly A (+) RNA was isolated by an oligo dT column (Aviv and Leder, 1972). Ten to 30 µg of total RNA was electrophoresed on a denaturing 1% agarose gel containing 2.2 M formaldehyde and transferred to nitrocellulose or Gene Screen (NEN Research Products) (Thomas, 1980). Alternately, 10 µg of total RNA was transferred directly to nitrocellulose using a slot blot technique. The membranes were hybridized with ^{32}P-labelled cDNA probe at 42°C in a solution of 50% formamide/5 x Denhardt's/0.1% SDS/100 µg/ml denatured salmon sperm DNA/0.9 M NcCl/50 mM sodium phosphate/5 mM EDTA (pH 7.4). After hybridization, the membranes were washed at room temperature in 0.3 M NaCl/30 mM trisodium citrate (pH 7.0) followed by washes at 45°C in 15 mM NaCl/1.5 mM trisodium citrate/0.1% SDS. Autoradiography was performed for 48-72 hours at -70°C.

Equal loading and transfer of the RNA samples was confirmed by acridine orange staining of the gel prior to and following transfer. As a further indicator of RNA quality, membranes were subsequently probed for actin, estrogen receptor, or progesterone receptor messages.

In Vitro Drug Sensitivity Assays

Tumor specimens were tested for resistance to either vinblastine or adriamycin using either the clonogenic assay or the MINI assay, both of which have been fully described elsewhere (Von Hoff et al., 1983; Kern et al., 1985). In brief, a single cell suspension derived from tumor material is exposed to the antineoplastic agent for one hour and then plated on agar. Sensitivity is defined as either < 50% tumor colony formation on day 14 (Von Hoff, 1983) or < 20% thymidine incorporation on day 3 (Kern, 1985) as compared to control plates with untreated tumor cell suspensions.

RESULTS

P-Glycoprotein Gene Amplification

A total of 275 breast cancer specimens and 33 specimens of other human cancers were hybridized on Southern blots with the P-glycoprotein cDNA probes. The same restriction fragments were detected by probes of both hamster and human origin (Fuqua et al., 1987). Twenty-two specimens of locally advanced disease and seven of metastatic breast cancer were obtained within three months after treatment with adriamycin, and thus were examples of clinically resistant disease. Another 21 breast cancer specimens and 22 cancers of other types were resistant to either adriamycin or vinblastine in the clonogenic or MINI assays. Surprisingly, as shown in Tables 1 and 2, there were no examples of P-glycoprotein gene amplification in any of these 308 human tumor specimens. Moreover, there were no instances of P-glycoprotein gene rearrangements.

TABLE 1. P-Glycoprotein Gene Amplification in Clinical Breast Cancer

	Amplified/Total
Stage I or II, Untreated	0/219
Locally advanced, after induction chemotherapy	0/22
Metastatic, after adriamycin	0/7
Total	0/248

Southern blots were reprobed for the actin gene, and these autoradiograms compared by densitometry with the autoradiograms obtained with the P-glycoprotein probe. This comparison demonstrated that any observed differences in P-glycoprotein signal were due to minor variations between specimens in the amount of DNA present (Merkel et al., 1987). In contrast, 30-fold P-glycoprotein gene amplification could be demonstrated in the MDA-A1 cell line by dilution analysis (Fuqua et al., 1987).

TABLE 2. P-Glycoprotein Gene Amplification and In Vitro Resistance to Adriamycin or Vinblastine

Tumor Type	Resistant	Sensitive	Amplified/Total
Breast	21	6	0/27
Sarcoma	3	5	0/8
Colon	3	2	0/5
Ovary	4	0	0/4
Stomach	4	0	0/4
Miscellaneous	8	4	0/12

P-Glycoprotein mRNA Expression

Since the P-glycoprotein gene can be overexpressed by some cell lines in the absence of, or prior to, gene amplification, we also examined many of these same tumors for mRNA overexpression with the P-glycoprotein cDNA probes. RNA from a total of 95 breast cancer specimens was studied, including 13 tumors with evidence of clinical resistance (defined above) and 16 tumors with in vitro resistance. As can be seen in Table 3, overexpression of P-glycoprotein message was not found in any specimen. In two cases of locally advanced disease, preparation of poly A (+) RNA was possible, and again P-glycoprotein message appeared to be absent (unpublished data).

TABLE 3. P-Glycoprotein mRNA Expression in Breast Cancer

Sample Characteristics	Overexpressed/Total
Stage I or II, Untreated	0/62
Stage III or IV, recently treated	0/13
Sensitive in vitro	0/4
Resistant in vitro	0/16

Overexpression of P-glycoprotein mRNA was invariably detected in RNA preparations from either the CHO-C5 or MDA-A1 cell lines, which were included as positive controls on each slot blot or Northern blot. In addition, P-glycoprotein mRNA was detected in a slot blot containing 10 μg of total RNA extracted from normal human kidney tissue, confirming the results of Fojo et al. (1987) and the sensitivity of our assay. Successful extraction and transfer of intact RNA from clinical samples was confirmed by the subsequent detection of messages for actin, estrogen receptor, and progesterone receptor by hybridization of the same blots with appropriate cDNA probes.

DISCUSSION

Our initial experience in generating a human MDR breast cancer cell line, marked by both overexpression and amplification of the P-glycoprotein gene, encouraged our search for a parallel mechanism of drug resistance in clinical breast cancer specimens. Such a finding would have important practical implications, since both adriamycin and vinca alkyloids are frequently employed in the treatment of this disease. Yet, in a large number of specimens of both untreated and resistant breast cancer, we found that the P-glycoprotein gene was neither amplified nor overexpressed. Clearly, the continuous process of stepwise selection to which MDR cell lines are exposed differs from the episodic exposure of clinical tumors to chemotherapy. Beyond this observation, other considerations are suggested by our findings regarding the P-glycoprotein gene in breast cancer.

Overexpression of P-glycoprotein mRNA has been detected in pheochromocytomas, neuroblastoma, colon cancer, and kidney cancer (Foto et al., 1987). The same group also reported that P-glycoprotein mRNA was overexpressed in normal adrenal, colon, kidney, and liver tissue. In contrast, only "low level" expression was found in other tumors, including breast cancer. There is evidence that the overexpression of P-glycoprotein may be one aspect of a multifaceted response to xenobiotics. This coordinate response, consisting of a decrease in cytochrome p450 activity, increase in anionic glutathione transferase, and expression of P-glycoprotein, has been observed in cell lines, regenerating or neoplastic liver tissue, and colon cancer (Thorgeirsson et al., 1987; Cowan et al., 1986; Batist et al., 1987). It is entirely conceivable that these phenotypic changes are limited in vivo to certain tissues. Tumors arising from these same tissues may consequently be more likely to display MDR than other tumors in which this response was not part of the premalignant repetoire.

These studies were performed on DNA or RNA which was isolated from tumors after homogenization. This approach cannot exclude the possible existence of small tumor subpopulations in which the P-glycoprotein gene is amplified overexpressed. Sensitive assays using in situ RNA hybridization would be required to exclude this possibility. Alternately, monoclonal antibodies directed against the P-glycoprotein could be used to detect MDR tumor subpopulations by immunohistochemistry or flow cytometry (Shenkenberg et al., 1986). Resistant subpopulations could grow out after drug exposure in a clonogenic assay, perhaps explaining some of the discrepancy between results of P-glycoprotein and clonogenic assays seen in Tables 2 and 3.

Nevertheless, these results provide strong evidence that the P-glycoprotein is unlikely to be responsible for most cases of primary adriamycin resistance in breast cancer. No more than 40% of previously untreated breast cancers will respond to adriamycin when given as a single agent (Tormey, 1975), yet amplification or overexpression of the P-glycoprotein gene was absent in all specimens of primary untreated breast cancer tested. In the same manner, P-glycoprotein is unlikely to contribute significantly to the frequent occurrence of acquired drug resistance in breast cancer. This gene was neither amplified nor overexpressed in specimens obtained shortly after adriamycin therapy, when most remaining cells could be expected to be clinically resistant.

These studies have immediate complications. Strategies to specifically overcome P-glycoprotein-mediated resistance to adriamycin are unlikely to be effective in breast cancer. A similar approach has already been attempted in ovarian cancer patients without success (Ozols et al., 1987). Secondly, attempts to target or image breast cancer cells with radiolabeled anti-P-glycoprotein monoclonal antibodies may not be successful. Finally, techniques such as those presented here will not be useful in predicting clinical drug resistance in breast cancer.

Though P-glycoprotein does not appear to be an important cause of drug resistance in breast cancer, it may, nontheless, play a central role in the resistance manifested by other malignancies. A number of other mechanisms of drug resistance have been delineated in cell lines. Among these are increased expression of anionic glutathione transferase and sorcin, and alterations in the cellular targets of various antineoplastic agents (Batist et al., 1986; Meyers and Biedler, 1987; Danks et al., 1987). Evidence must now be sought in human tumors that these mechanisms are active in vivo, as well as in vitro. The ability to detect alterations in the function of specific genes in clinical specimens may yet lead to accurate prediction of clinical drug resistance.

REFERENCES

Ling V (1975). Drug resistance and membrane alterations in mutants of mammalian cells. Can J Genet Cytol 17:503-515.

Juliano RL, Ling V (1976). A surface glycoprotein modulating drug permeability in Chinese hamster ovary cell mutants. Biochim Biophys Acta 455:152-162.

Ling V, Thompson LH (1974). Reduced permeability in CHO cells as a mechanism of resistance to colchicine. J Cell Physiol 83:103-116.

Beck WT, Mueller TJ, Tanzer LR (1979). Altered surface membrane glycoproteins in vinca alkyloid resistant human leukemic lymphoblasts. Cancer Res 39:2070-2076.

Akiyama S-I, Pastan I, Gottesman MD (1983). Isolation of human cell lines resistant to multiple drugs. J Cell Biol, 197-218a.

Dalton WS, Durie BGM, Alberts DS, Gerlach JH, Cress AE (1986). Characterization of a new drug-resistant myeloma cell line that expresses P-glycoprotein. Cancer Res 46:5125-5130.

Twentyman PR, Fox NE, Wright KA, Bleehen NM (1986). Derivation and preliminary characterization of adriamycin resistant lines of human lung cancer cells. Br J Cancer 53:529-537.

Tsuruo T, Iida H, Tsukagoshi S, Sakurai Y (1982). Increased accumulation of vincristine and adriamycin in drug-resistant P388 tumor cells following incubation with calcium antagonists and calmodulin inhibitors. Cancer Res 42:4730-4733.

Rogan AM, Hamilton TC, Young RC (1984). Reversal of adriamycin resistance by verapamil in human ovarian cancer. Science 224:994-996.

Willingham MC, Cornwell MM, Cardarelli CO, Gottesman MM, Pastran I (1986). Single cell analysis of daunomycin uptake and efflux in multidrug-resistant and -sensitive KB cells: Effects of verapamil and other drugs. Cancer Res 46:5941-5946.

Safa AR, Glover CJ, Averbuch SD, Meyers MB, Biedler JL, Felsted RL (1986). Photoaffinity labeling of membranes from sensitive and multidrug-resistant tumor cells with photoactive analogs of vinblastine. Proc Am Assoc Cancer Res, Abstract 1571, 396.

Hamada H, Tsuruo T (1986). Functional role for the 170- to 180-

kDa glycoprotein specific to drug resistant tumor cells as revealed by monoclonal antibodies. Proc Natl Acad Sci USA 83:7785-7789.

Gros P, Croop J, Housman D (1986). Mammalian multidrug resistance gene: Complete cDNA sequence indicates strong homology to bacterial transport proteins. Cell 47:371-380.

Chen C-J, Chin JE, Ueda K, Clark DP, Pastan I, Gottesman MM, Roninson RB (1986). Internal duplication and homology with bacterial transport proteins in the mdr1 (P-glycoprotein) gene from multidrug-resistant human cells. Cell 47:381-389.

Roninson IB, Chin JE, Choi KG, Gros P, Housman DE, Fojo A, Shen DW, Gottesman MM, Pastan I (1986). Isolation of human mdr DNA sequences amplified in multidrug-resistant KB carcinoma cells. Proc Natl Acad Sci USA 83:4538-4542.

Riordan JR, Deuchars K, Kartner N, Alon N, Trent J, Ling V (1985). Amplification of P-glycoprotein genes in multidrug-resistant mammalian cell lines. Nature 316:817-819.

Scotto KW, Biedler JL, Melera PW (1986). Amplification and expression of genes associated with multidrug resistance in mammalian cells. Science 232:751-755.

Gros P, Merish YB, Croop JM, Housman DE (1986). Isolation and expression of complementary DNA that confers multidrug resistance. Nature 323:728-731.

Roninson IB, Abelson HT, Housman DE, Howell N, Varshavsky A (1984). Amplification of specific DNA sequences correlates with multidrug resistance in Chinese hamster cells. Nature 309:626-628.

Gros P, Croop J, Roninson I, Varshavsky A, Housman DE (1986). Isolation and characterization of DNA sequences amplified in multidrug-resistant hamster cells. Proc Natl Acad Sci USA 83:337-341.

Fojo AT, Ueda K, Slamon DJ, Poplack DG, Gottesman MM, Pastan I (1987). Expression of a multidrug-resistance gene in human tumors and tissues. Proc Natl Acad Sci USA 84:265-269.

Gerlach JN, Bell DR, Karabousis C, Slocum HK, Kartner N, Tustum YM, Ling V, Baker RM (in press). P-glycoprotein in human sarcoma: Evidence for multidrug resistance. Clin Oncol.

Bell DR, Gerlach JH, Kartner N, Buick RN, Ling V (1985). Detection of P-glycoprotein in ovarian cancer: A molecular marker associated with multidrug resistance. J Clin Oncol 3:311-315.

Von Hoff DD, Clark GM, Stogdill BJ, Sarosday MF, O'Brien MT, Casper JT, Mattox DE, Page CP, Cruz AB, Sandbeck JF

(1983). Prospective clinical trial of a human tumor cloning system. Cancer Res 43:1926-1931.

Kern DH, Drogemuller CR, Kennedy MC, Hildebrand-Zanki SU, Tanigwa N, Sondak VK (1985). Development of a miniaturized, improved nucleic acid precursor incorporation assay for chemosensitivity testing of human solid tumors. Cancer Res 45:5436-5441.

Lathan B, Edwards DP, Dressler LG, Von Hoff DD, McGuire WL (1985). Immunological detection of Chinese hamster ovary cells expressing a multidrug resistance phenotype. Cancer Res 45:5064-5069.

Fuqua SAW, Moretti-Rojas IM, Schneider SL, McGuire WL (1987). P-glycoprotein expression in human breast cancer cells. Cancer Res 47:2103-2106.

Merkel DE, Fuqua SAW, Hill SM, Slamon D, Buzdar AU, McGuire WL (1987). Absence of P-glycoprotein gene amplification or overexpression in clinical breast cancer. Submitted for publication.

Young RA, Davis RW (1983). Efficient isolation of genes by using antibody probes. Proc Natl Acad Sci USA 80:1194-1198.

Maniatis T, Fritsch EF, Sambrook J (1982). "Molecular Cloning: A Laboratory Manual." Cold Spring Harbor: Cold Spring Harbor Laboratory.

Hortobagyi GN, Blumenstein GT, Spanos W, Montague ED, Buzdar AU, Yap H-Y, Schell F (1983). Multimodal treatment of locoregionally advanced breast cancer. Cancer 51:763-768.

Krieg P, Antmann E, Sauer G (1983). The simultaneous extraction of high-molecular-weight DNA and of RNA from solid tumors. Anal Biochem 134:288-294.

Giles KW, Meyers A (1965). An improved diphenylamine method for the estimation of deoxyribonucleic acid. Nature 206:93.

Southern EM (1975). Detection of specific sequences among DNA fragments separated by gel electrophoresis. J Mol Biol 98:503-517.

Glisin V, Crkenjakov R, Byres C (1974). Ribonucleic acid isolated by cesium chloride centrifugation. Biochemistry 13:2633-2637.

Aviv H, Leder P (1972). Purification of biologically active globin messenger RNA by chromatography on oligothymidylic acid-cellulose. Proc Natl Acad Sci USA 69:1408-1412.

Thomas P (1980). Hybridization of denatured RNA and small DNA fragments transferred to nitrocellulose. Proc Natl Acad Sci USA 77:5201.

Fuqua SAW, Dimas C, Von Hoff DD, Kern DH, McGuire WL (1987). P-glycoprotein amplification and expression fails to predict the chemosensitivity of human tumors in soft agar.

Submitted for publication.

Thorgeirsson SS, Huber BE, Sorrell S, Fojo A, Pastan I, Gottesman MM (1987). Expression of the multidrug-resistant gene in hepatocarcinogenesis and regenerating rat liver. Science 236:1120-1122.

Cowan KH, Batist G, Tulpule A, Sinha BK, Myers CE (1986). Similar biochemical changes associated with multidrug resistance in human breast cancer cells and carcinogen-induced resistance to xenobiotics in rats. Proc Natl Acad Sci USA 83:9328-9332.

Batist G, Hudson N, Mekhail-Ishak K, DeMuys JM (1987). Human colon cancer has the same biochemical phenotype as resistant carcinogen-induced preneoplastic nodules and as human breast cancer cells with multi-drug resistance (MDR). Proc Am Assoc Cancer Res, Abstract 1105, 279.

Shenkenberg T, Deacon T, Dressler LG, Von Hoff DD, McGuire WL (1986). Increase in drug resistance in CHO cells by enriching for P-glycoprotein by flow cytometry. Proc Am Assoc Cancer Res, Abstract 1036, 261.

Tormey DC (1975). Adriamycin (NSC 123127) in breast cancer. An overview of studies. Cancer Treat Rep 6:319-327.

Ozols RF, Cunnion RE, Klecker WR Jr, Hamilton TC, Ostchega Y, Parrillo JE, Young RC (1987). Verapamil and adriamycin in the treatment of drug-resistant ovarian cancer patients. J Clin Oncol 5:641-647.

Batist G, Tulpule A, Sinha BK, Katki AG, Myers CE, Cowan KH (1986). Overexpression of a novel anionic glutathione transferase in multidrug-resistant human breast cancer cells. J Biol Chem 261:15544-15549.

Meyers MB, Biedler JL (1987). Possible role for sorcin, a calcium-binding protein overproduced in multidrug resistant (MDR) cells. Proc Am Assoc Cancer Res, Abstract 1148, 290.

Danks MK, Yalowich JC, Beck WT (1987). Atypical multiple drug resistance in a human leukemic cell line selection for resistance to teniposide (VM-26). Cancer Res 47:1297-1301.

Prediction of Response to Cancer Therapy, pages 75–92
© 1988 Alan R. Liss, Inc.

NON-CLONOGENIC, IN VITRO ASSAYS FOR PREDICTING
SENSITIVITY TO CANCER CHEMOTHERAPY[1]

Larry M. Weisenthal,[2] Yong-zhuang Su,
Thomas E. Duarte, and Robert A. Nagourney

Veterans Administration Medical Center, Long
Beach, CA (LMW and TED), University
of California, Irvine (LMW, YZS and RAN),
and Oncotech, Inc., Irvine, CA (RAN)

[1] Supported by the Veterans Administration,
Memorial Hospital Medical Center Foundation,
NIH 1R43CA43432-01 and Oncotech, Inc.

[2] Current address: Oncotech, Inc., 1791
Kaiser Avenue, Irvine, CA 92714, USA

INTRODUCTION

There have been many attempts to develop tests to
predict responses to anti-cancer drugs during the
past forty years (Black and Speer, 1954; Hanauske,
et al, 1985; Tanneberger and Nissen, 1983;
Weisenthal and Lippman, 1985). None of the many
proposed tests have achieved wide-spread
acceptance. A major problem is that almost all
fresh human tumor specimens contain large number
of normal cells, such as macrophages, white blood
cells, fibroblasts, and proliferating normal
epithelial cells (Smith, et al, 1985). The "human
tumor clonogenic" assay was alleged to circumvent
this problem by virtue of permitting only
selective growth of tumor cells. However, this
assay was not found to be practical and reliable
for most applications because clumps of cells and
debris could not be distinguished from true
colonies of cells, because there was inconsistent
growth of tumor cells, because the assay generally
required fourteen days for a result, and because

Table I Advantages and Disadvantages of
Predictive Cancer Chemosensitvity Assays

Theoretical(A)Advantage and(D)Disadvantage

Assay Type

Clonogenic

(A) Measures cells capable of several divisions

(A) Tumor response may be predicted by a mutiple log kill of clonogenic cells

(A) Cell cycle-specific agents may be tested in valid assays

(D) G_0 cells cannot be measured

Uptake of DNA precursors or precursor analogues(3H-thymidine, BUdR, etc.)

(A) Early inhibition of DNA synthesis may often be predictive of a multiple log kill of stem cells or clonogenic cells

(A) Cell cycle-specific agents may be tested in valid assays

(D) G_0 cells cannot be measured

Sub-renal capsule

(A) Early evidence of cell lysis may often be predictive of a multiple log kill of stem cells or clonogenic cells

(A) 3-dimensional tumor architecture maintained; drug biotransformation and host toxicity more realistically modeled than with *in vitro* assays

(A) G_0 cells are measured

(D) Cycle-specific drugs may be inadequately tested

Differential Staining Cytotoxicity (**DISC**) Assay

(A) Early evidence of cell damage may often predict for a multiple log kill of stem or clonogenic cells

(A) G_0 cells are measured

(D) Cycle-specific drugs may be inadequately tested

Table II Advantages and Disadvantages of Predictive Cancer Chemosensitvity Assays

Assay Type	Practical (A) Advantage and (D) Disadvantage
Clonogenic	(D) Results unavailable for 2 weeks or more
	(D) Unavoidable presence of cell clumps and poor growth of colonies make detection of multiple log cell kill impossible
	(D) Most assays are technically invalid due to poor growth and clumping
	(A) Many studies have reported positive clinical correlations and many laboratories are now familiar with the technology
Uptake of DNA precursors or precursor analogues (3H-thymidine, BUdR, etc.)	(D) Potential technical artifacts exist (DNA replication versus repair, alterations in DNA synthesis pathways and "pool" sizes, labeling of normal cells, etc.)
	(A) Assay not invalidated by clumps
	(A) Promising pilot data exist
Sub-renal capsule	(A) Highest evaluability rate of all assays reported to date
	(D) "Growth" may be due to inflammation, while "shrinkage" may be due to a necrotic portion of specimen
	(D) Expense and inconvenience of mice
	(A) Promising pilot data
Differential Staining Cytotoxicity (DiSC) Assay	(A) High evaluability rate, specific for tumor cells, not invalidated by presence of clumps (few artifacts)
	(A) Can test many drugs from a small specimen
	(D) Requires skilled technologist to recognize and count tumor cells, tedious
	(A) Promising pilot data, especially in hematologic neoplasms

the assay required large numbers of cells, making it difficult to test enough drugs and drug concentrations to yield useful information. It is possible that future research may solve the above problems, but it is not clear that clonogenic assays are advantageous compared to more straightforward assays based upon measuring drug effects on the total tumor cell population (Weisenthal and Lippman, 1985, Tables 1 and 2). It is our opinion that currently existing, non-clonogenic assays may be usefully applied to address important questions in cancer therapy (Weisenthal, 1987). We will begin by discussing some theoretical considerations relating to assays which measure cell proliferation as compared to assays which do not measure cell proliferation. We will then proceed to describe how our laboratory has applied one particular type of non-proliferation assay as a tool to identify strategies for circumventing acquired drug resistance in human lymphatic neoplasms.

PROLIFERATION ASSAYS

It is an obvious observation that cancer produces morbidity and mortality as a consequence of cell proliferation. Additionally, the most common experimental models of cancer (i.e. established cell lines and transplantable rodent tumors) contain cell populations with very high growth fractions, frequently approaching 100%. It is, therefore, not surprising that most investigational chemosensitivity assays have utilized cell proliferation or DNA synthesis as the assay endpoint. In systems where the cell growth fraction approaches 100%, almost any type of endpoint will be reflective of changes in cell proliferation and will usually correlate nicely with the changes in the surviving cell fraction, after appropriate assay calibration. As listed in Table III, common methods for measuring differences in cell proliferation in systems with high cell growth fractions have included (1) counting cells several generation times following drug exposure (by a variety of methods), (2) measuring total cell culture metabolism (by a variety of methods) and (3) estimating DNA synthesis using probes such as radioactive thymidine or BUdR.

Table III   Total Cell Proliferation Assays

In culture conditions where growth fraction approaches 100%

a.   Cell counting several generations times after drug exposure

      e.g. FACS, DiSC Assay, Coulter Counter, Image analysis of monolayers (e.g. Lifetrac), Spheroid sizing, Automated volume integration of soft agar colonies/clumps

b.   Measuring total cell culture metabolism several generation times after drug exposure

      e.g. succinate dehydrogenase (Tetrazolium, ATP, glycolysis [Bactec], etc.)

c.   DNA synthesis probes

      e.g. radioactive thymidine, BUdR

In tumor cell systems where the cell growth
fraction is low, total cell counts and metabolic
endpoints will not necessarily be reflective of
cell proliferation and a specific DNA synthesis
probe is needed, if an anti-proliferative endpoint
is desired. In a heterogeneous cell population
(such as that existing in most fresh human
neoplasms) a reliable system must also exist for
selectively eliminating or suppressing non-tumor
cells or else for selectively identifying tumor
cells. The presence and growth of normal
epithelial cells (Smith, et al, 1985), connective
tissue cells, and inflammatory cells in cultures
of fresh human neoplasms is a problem which
continues to be underappreciated in the current
chemosensitivity assay literature. Though widely
used, proliferation assays do not measure the
chemosensitivity of non-cycling cells, which may
be an important determinant of long or medium-term
response. These assays are also of limited use in
neoplasms such as CLL, where the fraction of
cycling cells is very small and difficult to
identify.

NON-PROLIFERATION ASSAYS

There are an increasing number of
non-proliferation assays currently being applied
to fresh human tumors with low growth fractions.
Some examples of these non-proliferation assays
are listed in Table IV.

The biological relevance of these
non-proliferation assays is frequently not
appreciated. A theoretical argument favoring the

*Table IV. Non-Proliferation Assays in Cells with
a Low Growth Fraction*

1. Cell Metabolism

   ATP
   Bactec
   Tetrazolium

2. Membrane integrity

   DiSC, trypan blue, ethidium bromide, etc.
   Fluorescein Diacetate (by FACS or "Rotman")
   Radiolabeled chromium release
   Monolayer adherence

3. Morphology (pyknosis, etc.)

4. Resistance Loci

   Steroid receptors
   GP-170 protein, gene copies and transcripts
   DHFR levels or DHFR gene copies
   Other target enzymes or inactivation enzymes
   Intracellular drug accumulation
   GSH levels

utilization of non-proliferation assays is the
possibility that temporarily non-cycling tumor
cells may be important targets for cancer therapy
and, yet, are not measured by cell proliferation
assays. A potential criticism of
non-proliferation assays is that some forms of
cancer therapy (notably radiation and
cycle-specific drugs) may be effective largely
through a cytostatic mechanism, while having
little direct effect on overall cell metabolism or

membrane integrity. For this latter reason, non-proliferation assays are often dismissed without proper consideration.

We will now attempt to consider the following theoretical question: *Are non-proliferation assays measuring short-term changes induced by drugs capable of distinguishing between drug-sensitive and drug-resistant cell populations?* The answer to this question is clearly *yes*, provided that the mechanism of early cell damage measured by the assay is related to the mechanism of cytotoxicity in vivo. The answer to this question is also *yes*, even is the mechanism of early cell damage measured by the assay in vitro is unrelated to the mechanism of cytotoxicity in vivo, *provided that* the mechanism of drug resistance in vitro is related to the mechanism of resistance in vivo (this point will be illustrated below). However, short-term, non-proliferation assays may *not* accurately reflect the state of drug resistance if the mechanism of early cell damage in vitro is unrelated to the mechanism of cytotoxicity in vivo and the mechanism of resistance in vitro is unrelated to the mechanism of resistance in vivo.

Figure 1 illustrates an example of how the mechanism of in vitro toxicity may be different than the mechanism of in vivo toxicity, yet the mechanisms of in vitro and in vivo resistance may be the same. Many drugs work by binding to DNA and/or interfering with DNA function. Cells attempt to protect themselves by excising damaged DNA and repairing this DNA damage. In vivo, at low drug concentrations, the results of inadequate repair is division-linked cell death. In vitro, in situations where cells are not dividing, cell death may occur in the absence of cell division by a previously-described suicide pathway in which excess DNA excision or else slow repair results in

Mechanisms of In Vitro Toxicity May be Different than In Vivo Toxicity, but Mechanisms of Resistance may be the Same.

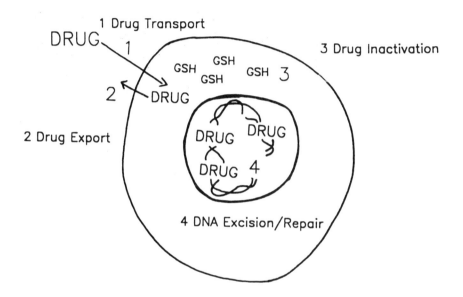

In Vitro—"High" drug concentration

Result of excess excision or slow repair is increased synthesis of poly—ADP—ribose which results in decreased NAD, ATP, glycolysis and cell death.

In Vivo—"Low" drug concentration

Result of inadequate repair is division—linked cell death.

Figure 1

increased synthesis of poly-ADP-ribose, which
results in decreased cellular NAD, ATP,
glycolysis, and cell death *not* linked to cell
division (Carson, et al, 1986; Berger, 1985;
Whish, et al, 1975). Even though the mechanisms
of cell killing may be different in dividing cells
and non-dividing cells, the mechanisms of
resistance may be the same, as depicted here. For
example, resistant cells may exhibit defective
drug transport into the cell, enhanced drug export
out of the cell, enhanced drug inactivation
through drug metabolism or glutathione, or else
rapid and efficient excision/repair. By testing
non-proliferating cells in vitro at
appropriately-calibrated drug concentrations, one
may be very good at accurately discriminating
between cells with varying degrees of drug
resistance. More importantly, one may then go on
to utilize the assay system to identify successful
strategies for circumventing drug resistance in
clinical neoplasms.

USE OF A NON-PROLIFERATION ASSAY TO STUDY THE
CIRCUMVENTION OF DRUG RESISTANCE IN HUMAN
LYMPHATIC NEOPLASMS

We have previously described and tested the
Differential Staining Cytotoxicity (DiSC)
chemosensitivity assay in human lymphatic
neoplasms (Weisenthal, et al, 1986). This assay
was found to accurately detect acquired drug
resistance in acute lymphoblastic leukemia and in
chronic lymphocytic leukemia. First, the activity
spectrum of standard drugs in vitro was found to
correspond well with the known clinical activity
spectrum of these agents. Second, there were good
prospective clinical correlations with in vitro
assay results in individual patients. Third,
cells from previously-treated patients were
significantly more resistant in vitro than were
cells from previously-untreated patients. Fourth,

with repeated assays performed over time on cells
from the same patients, there was increasing in
vitro resistance in the presence of intravening
chemotherapy but no significant change in the
absence of intravening chemotherapy.
Collectively, the preceding data provided
compelling evidence for the accuracy of the assay
in discriminating between drug resistant and drug
sensitive cell populations in human lymphatic
neoplasms.

Figure 2 shows results from 47 assays on cells
from different patients with acute lymphoblastic
leukemia tested with vincristine. On the Y axis
is plotted percent cell survival. 100% cell
survival indicates 0% cell kill or the absence of
drug effect. 0% cell survival indicates complete
tumor cell kill. The X axis indicates the
chemosensitivity percentile of assays on cells
from individual patients. A specimen in the 95th
percentile would be more sensitive to vincristine
than 95% of all similar specimens. A specimen in
the 50th percentile would be more sensitive than
half the specimens and more resistant than the
other half. A specimen in the 10th percentile
would be more resistant than 90% of the specimens
of the same type, and so on. In this graph, we
show the respective plots of assays performed on
cells from either previously-untreated patients or
else from relapsed patients. A similar plot of
assay results from untreated patients with acute
non-lymphoblastic leukemia is shown for
comparison. It can be seen that specimens from
relapsed patients were dramatically and
significantly more resistant in the DiSC assay
than were specimens from previously-untreated
patients. With this work, we have defined percent
cell survivals and confidence limits that are
characteristic of untreated patients (26 +/- 4.5,
N = 22) and relapsed patients (62 +/- 4.8, N =
25), respectively. We hypothesize that an active
resistance-modification agent would change the in

Figure 2

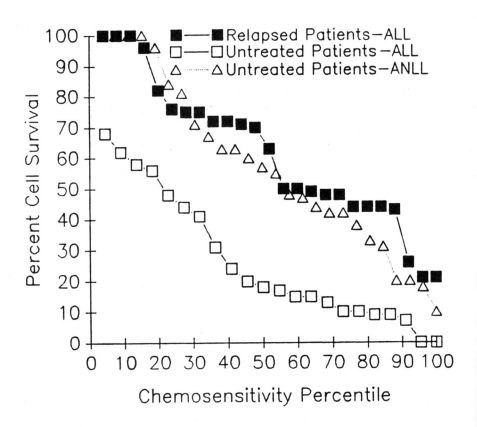

vitro chemosensitivity of specimens from relapsed patients to the range observed in specimens from previously-untreated patients. Results using this approach are described below. In contrast with virtually all other systems for studying acquired drug resistance, the DiSC assay system accurately reflects drug resistance in fresh cells from human patients, as resistance acquired in the course of clinical chemotherapy, not as derived from artificial laboratory passage of cells in the presence of increasing drug concentrations.

The following are potential strategies for circumventing acquired drug resistance in human lymphatic neoplasms identified through the use of the DiSC assay. First, menadiol (Vitamin K_3) was found to selectively enhance the activity of a number of standard drugs in resistant tumor specimens (Su, et al, 1987). Second, Nagourney and colleagues reported that buthionine sulfoximine selectively potentiated nitrogen mustard in drug-resistant specimens of chronic lymphocytic leukemia (Nagourney, et al, 1987). Thirdly, as described below, the combination of verapamil and lidocaine, at clinically-achievable concentrations, selectively reversed resistance to vincristine and doxorubicin in assays performed in fresh specimens of ALL, CLL, lymphoma and multiple myeloma.

We began by screening 6 putative protein kinase C antagonists, tested together at fixed, clinically achievable concentrations. The agents tested and concentrations (in ug/ml) included verapamil (0.5), imipramine (0.5), lidocaine (6.0), tamoxifen (0.15), chlorpromazine (0.75), and haloperidol (0.1). (This complex combination is hereafter referred to as VILTCH). When the VILTCH combination was tested alone in fresh specimens of ALL, there was minimal toxicity (Figure 3). This was not entirely unexpected as both phenothiazines (Borsa, et al, 1986) and lidocaine (Chlebowski, et

Figure 3

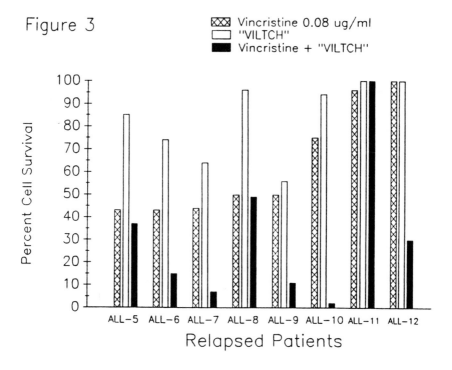

Vincristine 0.08 ug/ml
"VILTCH"
Vincristine + "VILTCH"

Relapsed Patients

Figure 4

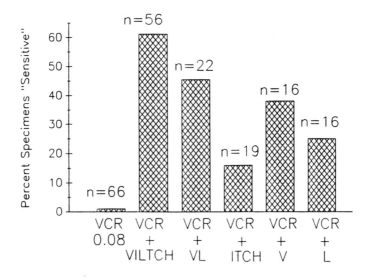

al, 1982) have previously been shown to have a degree of toxicity to established tumor cell lines. When VILTCH was tested in combination with vincristine in 4 specimens of previously-untreated ALL, results compared to vincristine alone were no different in 3 cases and additive in 1 case. In contrast, when VILTCH was tested in specimens from relapsed patients (Figure 3), there was no effect in 3 cases (patients #5, 8, and 11) but clear synergy in 5 other cases (patients #6, 7, 9, 10, and 12). In all 8 of the assays performed on cells from relapsed patients, the percent cell survival to vincristine alone was well above the mean range (26 =/- 4.5, Fig. 2) characteristic of the drug-sensitive specimens of previously-untreated patients. However, in 62% (5/8) of the assays, VILTCH converted the percent cell survivals from the range characteristic of relapsed patients to range characteristic of previously-untreated patients (Figure 3).

In order to determine which drugs in the VILTCH combination were most active in reversing resistance to vincristine, additional work was carried out in chronic lymphocytic leukemia (CLL), a neoplasm more readily available for study at our institution. Figure 4 shows that 66 specimens of CLL were resistant (cell survival greater than 30%) to vincristine alone in the DiSC assay. The addition of VILTCH converted about 60% of the assays to a "sensitive" range. The four drug combination "ITCH" was effective only about 15% of the time, while verapamil and lidocaine (singly and especially in combination) appeared to be the most important components of the VILTCH combination. It should again be noted that the concentrations of verapamil and lidocaine tested here fall definitely within the clinically achievable range, as contrasted with previously published results in other systems, where generally toxic concentrations of verapamil have been tested. The 2 drug combination of verapamil and lidocaine is theoretically attractive from a clinical point of view, as these agents have very different effects on myocardial conductivity and would not be expected to exhibit additive toxicity if used together. Thus, the use of these agents in combination could provide greater assurance that therapeutically effective levels of at least one agent could be maintained at all times during treatment with the chemotherapeutic regimen. We are currently carrying out clinical trials to evaluate the clinical efficacy of verapamil + lidocaine in restoring drug sensitivity in human patients with acquired drug resistance.

In conclusion, the non-clonogenic, non-proliferation DiSC chemosensitivity assay accurately discriminates between drug sensitive and drug resistant cell populations from fresh specimens of human lymphatic neoplasms. This assay may be utilized to identify strategies for circumventing drug resistance in human lymphatic neoplasms. Clinical trials should soon indicate whether or not anti-resistance strategies identified through the use of non-clonogenic assays are efficacious.

REFERENCES

Berger, NA. Poly (ADP-ribose) in the cellular response to DNA damage. Radiat Res 101:4-15, 1985

Black, MM and Speer, FD. Further observations on the effects of cancer chemotherapeutic agents on the in vitro dehydrogenase activity of cancer tissue. J Natl Cancer Inst 14:1147-58, 1954

Borsa, J, Einspenner, M, Sargent, MD, and Hickie, RA. Selective cytotoxicity of calmidazolium and trifluoperazine for cycling versus non-cycling C3H10T1/2 cells in vitro. Cancer Res 46:133-36. 1986

Carson, DA, Seto, S, Wasson, DB, and Carrera, CJ. DNA strand breaks, NAD metabolism, and programmed cell death. Exptl Cell Res 164:273-81, 1986

Chlebowski, RT, Block, JB, Cundiff, D, and Dietrich, MF. Doxorubicin cytotoxicity enhanced by local anesthetics in a human melanoma cell line. Cancer Treat Rep 66:121-25, 1982

Hanauske, AR, Hanauske, U, and Von Hoff, DD. The human tumor cloning assay in cancer research and therapy: a review with clinical correlations. Curr Probl Cancer 9:1-50, 1985

Nagourney, RA, Messenger, JC, and Evans, S. In vitro perturbations in nitrogen mustard sensitivity in primary cultures of benign and malignant human lymphocytes induced by L-2-oxothiazolidine-4-carboxylate (OTZ) and buthionine sulfoximine (BSO). Proc AM Assoc Cancer Res 28:284, 1987

Smith, HS, Lippman, ME, Hiller, AJ et al. Response to adriamycin of cultured normal and malignant human mammary epithelial cells. J Natl Cancer Inst 74:341-7, 1985

Su, YZ, Duarte, TE, Dill, PL, and Weisenthal, LM. Selective enhancement by menadiol of in vitro drug activity in human lymphatic neoplasms. Cancer Treat Rep 71:619-625, 1987

Tanneberger, S and Nissen, E. Predicting response of human solid tumors to chemotherapy. Cancer Treat Rev 10:203-219, 1983

Weisenthal, LM. Clones, dyes, nuclides, mouse kidneys, and ...virions: a new-non-clonogenic assay for tumor chemosensitivity. Eur J Cancer Clin Oncol 23:9-12, 1987

Weisenthal, LM, Dill, PL, Finklestein, JZ, Duarte, TE, Baker, JA, and Moran, EM. Laboratory detection of primary and acquired drug resistance in human lymphatic neoplasms. Cancer Treat Rep 70:1283-95, 1986

Weisenthal, LM, and Lippman, ME. Clonogenic and non-clonogenic in vitro chemosensitivity assays. Cancer Treat Rep 69:615-32, 1985

Whish, WJD, Davies, MI, and Shall, S. Stimulation of poly (ADP-ribose) polymerase activity by the anti-tumor antibiotic, streptozotocin. Biochem Biophys Res Comm 65:722-730, 1975

Prediction of Response to Cancer Therapy, pages 93–103
© 1988 Alan R. Liss, Inc.

INHIBITION OF DNA SYNTHESIS IN SELECTION OF ANTICANCER THERAPY

Rosella Silvestrini, Ornella Sanfilippo, Maria Grazia Daidone and Nadia Zaffaroni

Oncologia Sperimentale C, Istituto Nazionale per lo Studio e la Cura dei Tumori, Via Venezian 1, 20133 Milan, Italy

INTRODUCTION

Clinical evidence has unequivocally shown that human tumors display a drug responsiveness quite different from that of experimental tumors. A high intertumor heterogeneity in response to drugs characterizes the different human tumor types, and it can be stated that there are no sensitive or resistant histotypes, but only histotypes more or less sensitive or resistant to drugs.

The variability in response to drugs by tumors clinically similar and the general decrease in drug sensitivity with progression of the disease, as a likely age-dependent phenomenon, have prompted the design of suitable systems for a taylored therapy or for basic and clinically oriented studies on human tumors.

The first aim has met many limitations in its clinical use and has been largely restricted to the management of heavily pretreated or naturally resistant tumors. A prospective study on adequate and homogeneous series of patients with sensitive or moderately sensitive tumor types has never been rigorously performed to define the role of in vitro chemosensitivity tests in selecting active drugs and in sparing toxic side effects by eliminating ineffective drugs.

The second aim, which has included genetic, biochemical and biologic investigations, has been recently extended to clinically oriented studies. An important potential of

in vitro sensitivity tests is the possibility to acquire
information to better understand whether or to what extent
the increased failure of response to chemotherapy with
progression of disease is actually due to the onset of cell
drug resistance, as hypothetically assumed (Goldie and
Coldman, 1979), or to a tumor burden greater than the
therapeutic potential of clinical treatment. An already
consolidated field of research is also represented by the
use of these experimental systems for in vitro phase II
studies on previously untreated tumors and for the knowledge of natural or induced coresistance among analogs or
unrelated drugs.

METHODOLOGIC ASPECTS

The in vitro systems which have been proposed and used
can be essentially grouped in three main categories according to the drug-effect target considered: clonogenic
assays, cytocidal assays (which evaluate cell viability,
suppression of DNA and protein synthesis, or inhibition of
respiration processes), and antimetabolic assays (based on
short-term incorporation of nucleic acid or protein-labeled
precursors). The initial discordance among results
obtained by the different systems markedly faded when
conditions specific for each assay, and mainly related to
drug concentrations and sensitivity criteria, were adopted
(Durie et al., 1982; Sanfilippo et al., 1984).

We have used for a decade a short-term antimetabolic
assay which evaluates the interference of drugs on the
incorporation of nucleic acid precursors. Since requisits
for basic and clinically oriented studies and for clinical
application are the handling and the reliability of the
system, we have performed a multistep verification to make
it as feasible, reliable and simple as possible. The main
methodologic aspects we investigated and defined were the
labeled precursor and drug concentration, the expression of
incorporation values for cell suspensions or solid samples,
and the criteria for definition of in vitro sensitivity.

As regards the first point, the pool equilibrating
concentrations of nucleic acid precursors were defined for
various tumor types. Analysis of the in vitro response
rate to single drugs performed on large series of several
tumor types has shown the concentrations defined according

to the formula of Tisman et al. (1973) as those able to reproduce the clinical response rates reported for the same drugs used in monochemotherapy for the different tumor types.

To make the test applicable also to fragments, total radioactivity incorporation was considered for homogeneous cell suspensions from systemic diseases, and fractional incorporation for fragments from solid tumors.

Finally, analysis of the relation between in vitro sensitivity and clinical response of individual tumors evidenced that short-term antimetabolic effects superior to the variation coefficient of control samples are indicative of clinical response. Anyway, inhibitions lower than 20%, which represents the median variation coefficient value recorded in control samples on large series of different tumor types, were not considered as a drug effect. Somewhat different sensitivity criteria were adopted only for a few drugs which exhibited high in vitro activities in some tumor types (Silvestrini et al., 1983).

The outcome of this multiple approach is a very simple test which consists of 3 h of in vitro treatment, with [^{3}H]thymidine labeling during the last hour. In fact, similar drug effects have been observed on [^{3}H]thymidine and [^{3}H]uridine incorporation in all the tumor types and for all the conventional drugs, so to justify consideration of only the DNA precursor. The main advantages are the short time (2 days), the relatively low cost and high technical simplicity. Moreover, the possibility to use solid samples avoids cell damage and bias due to disaggregation procedures and greatly increases the feasibility for all tumor types. The main limitations are the impossibility to detect long-term DNA repair and to test different treatment schedules.

FIELDS OF RESEARCH

An area in which the in vitro test has been extensively evaluated is individual tumor sensitivity to drugs used in clinical trials in view of the clinical application on individual patients. Clinical response to conventional drug combinations was analysed in relation to in vitro sensitivity to the same drugs tested individually on a series of 177 patients with different advanced tumor types.

Clinical treatment consisted mainly of PVB or PEB for testicular tumors, CVP $\sim$ ABP for non-Hodgkin lymphomas, AV for breast cancers, cisplatin for ovarian cancers, and dacarbazine for malignant melanomas. Retrospective analysis showed a generally high overall agreement between in vitro sensitivity and objective clinical response of individual tumors to the same drugs (Daidone et al., 1985; Sanfilippo et al., 1986; Silvestrini et al., 1985), which decreased with increasing resistance clinically attested for the different tumor types (Table 1). In fact, for the highly chemoresistant malignant melanomas an extremely poor agreement was observed. Similarly, the predictive accuracy in sensitivity reached very high values for germ cell testicular tumors and non-Hodgkin lymphomas, still remarkable values for breast and epithelial ovarian cancers, but dropped to a very low value for malignant melanomas. Conversely, the predictive accuracy in resistance is not apparently related to clinical resistance of different tumor types and other factors, such as the inability of the test to reproduce the additive or synergistic effect of drugs and the criteria for the evaluation of the clinical response, needed to be invoked.

Table 1. Relation between in vitro sensitivity and objective clinical response

	Type of lesion	Overall agreement (%)	True positive (%)	True negative (%)	P value
Testicular tumor*	Metastases	90	93	80	< 0.01
Non-Hodgkin lymphomas*		79	86	66	< 0.01
Breast cancers†	Primary	78	75	81	< 0.01
Ovarian cancers†	Metastases	68	78	64	< 0.05
Malignant melanomas†	Metastases	46	18	91	NS

* Complete response.
† Partial response $\geq$ 50%.

Some technical and biological aspects have been considered as potential responsible factors for the variable agreement rates between in vitro data and objective clinical response. An intrinsic limitation of a test which evaluates a short-term antimetabolic effect in detecting long-term damage repair was investigated. The in vitro activity of different drugs was evaluated with the short-term antimetabolic assay and with a cytocidal assay based on the inhibition of $[^3]$thymidine incorporation, in ovarian cancers and malignant melanomas (Zaffaroni et al., 1987). An overestimation of drug effect, limited to malignant melanomas, was observed by recording short-term metabolic perturbations in comparison to cytocidal effect. This finding is in agreement with the high rate of false positives observed for malignant melanomas by using the antimetabolic assay and could be explained by the important phenomenon of damage repair in clinically resistant tumors. Similarly, tumor burden greater than the therapeutic potential of clinical treatment could be responsible for the occurrence of in vitro false positives.

Another factor responsible for the predictive accuracy of in vitro tests is biologic interlesional heterogeneity, which makes the type of lesion tested in vitro extremely important (Von Hoff, 1985). The frequent availability of primary tumor material during surgery or the objective inaccessibility of metastatic lesions has practically led in the past to mainly consider primary lesions or all the lesions together. This point has been carefully investigated in germ cell testicular tumors and epithelial ovarian cancers (Table 2). We observed that the sensitivity of the primary tumor is a poor indicator of the objective clinical response evaluated on metastatic lesions after removal of the primary, whereas the in vitro drug sensitivity of metastatic lesions is highly and statistically correlated with objective clinical response.

However, a disagreement between in vitro and in vivo results is not necessarily ascribable to inaccuracy of in vitro testing, and the reliability of clinical response in reflecting biologic eradication of the disease may be questioned. In this regard, the predictivity of in vitro sensitivity or objective clinical response on long-term clinical outcome has been analyzed in patients with non-Hodgkin lymphomas (Table 3). The probability of 6-year survival was quite similar for patients for whom in vitro

Table 2. Predictivity of in vitro sensitivity on clinical response as a function of the tumor lesion tested in vitro

	Overall agreement (%)	True positive (%)	True negative (%)	P value
Ovarian cancers				
Primary	44	71	35	NS
Metastasis	68	78	64	<0.05
Testicular tumors				
Primary	65	100	14	NS
Metastasis	90	93	80	<0.01

Table 3. Long-term outcome as a function of in vitro sensitivity or objective clinical response in non-Hodgkin lymphomas*

	Probability of 6-year survival (%)
Clinical	
Responders	68
Nonresponders	10
In vitro	
Sensitive	66
Resistant	7

* Treatment: CVP ∿ ABP for most or miscellanea.

tumor drug sensitivity had been proved at a preclinical level and for patients who reached objective clinical response, which indicates the similar reliability of in vitro and in vivo findings, but with the advantage of obtaining information earlier with the first approach.

This result prompted an analysis of the prognostic relevance of in vitro sensitivity on long-term clinical outcome, irrespectively of its agreement with short-term objective clinical response (Table 4). In patients with locally advanced breast cancers treated with adriamycin and vincristine in between locoregional treatment (surgery or radiotherapy), the in vitro sensitivity was not related to freedom from progression or overall survival. The main limitation of this study was that in vitro sensitivity was determined on the primary lesion. In a more recent study on patients with advanced ovarian cancers, most of them treated with cisplatin and a few also with cyclophosphamide or doxorubicin, in vitro sensitivity of metastatic lesions to the same drugs was indicative of a significantly higher probability of freedom from progression but not of overall survival. Conversely, in patients with non-Hodgkin lymphomas at stages II, III and IV according to the Ann Arbor classification, treated with multidrug combinations, in vitro sensitivity evaluated on lymph node lesions was significantly correlated with probability of freedom from progression and overall survival.

Table 4. Long-term clinical outcome as a function of in vitro sensitivity (S) or resistance (R)

	Time (yr)	Probability (%) of					
		FFP*			Survival		
		S	R	p	S	R	p
Breast cancers	4	28	25	NS	54	55	NS
Ovarian cancers	1.5	44	22	0.057	58	72	NS
Non-Hodgkin lymphomas	6	26	6	<0.01	66	7	<0.01

* Freedom from progression

The cell kinetic variable has also been considered in view of the even more evident importance of the potential proliferative activity as a long-term predictor of biologic aggressiveness of the tumor (Del Bino et al., 1986) but not of sensitivity to drugs (Table 5). Cell kinetics gives no additional prognostic information on progression-free survival, but it represents a further determinant of survival in the subset of patients with in vitro-sensitive tumors. In addition, whereas patients with slowly proliferating, in vitro-sensitive tumors have a probability of about 80% to survive at 6 years, no patient with a fast-proliferating, in vitro-resistant tumor has any probability to be alive at that time.

Table 5. Clinical outcome as a function of cell kinetics and in vitro sensitivity in non-Hodgkin lymphomas

In vitro	Probability of 6-year FFP (%)			Survival (%)		
	Overall	Slow*	Fast	Overall	Slow	Fast
Sensitive	26	26	28	66	79	47
		NS			< 0.01	
Resistant	6	12	0	7	12.5	0
		NS			NS	

* Proliferative rate defined according to the median [^{3}H]thymidine labeling index.

These results suggest that the eventual prevalence or the onset of natural or induced chemoresistant cell subpopulations can compromise the long-term success of an in vitro test in the more clinically resistant ovarian cancers, but not in the more sensitive non-Hodgkin lymphomas. Preclinical chemosensitivity and cell proliferative rate appear to be two important prognostic factors, but with a modulation in their relative significance in the different tumor types.

Unfortunately, only retrospective studies on homogeneous series of patients or scanty prospective studies (Alberts et al., 1984; Meyskens et al., 1984; Von Hoff et al., 1983) are available. The precise role of in vitro tests in selecting active drugs and in excluding the ineffective and toxic ones at a preclinical level will be defined only by prospective trials which compare the efficacy of one or two in vitro-active drugs with conventional drug combinations.

In a study on patients with advanced germ cell testicular tumors at salvage or palliation chemotherapy, we used the in vitro assay for conventional drugs to plan individual patient treatment (Table 6). About half of the patients were treated with in vitro inactive drugs because of a general resistance to all the tested drugs. A significantly poorer response for all the clinical endpoints considered was observed for patients treated with in vitro inactive drugs than for those treated with active drugs. This result further supports the reliability of the in vitro evaluation of cell sensitivity in reproducing clinical responsiveness.

Table 6. Clinical response in patients with testicular tumors treated with assay-directed therapy

In vitro	Objective response (%)*	FFP (%)[†]	Survival (%)[†]
Sensitive	54	27	36
	p = 0.02	p<0.01	p < 0.01
Resistant	10	0	0

* Partial response $\geq$ 50%.
[†] At 26 months.

Finally, the antimetabolic in vitro assay has been used for important basic and clinically oriented studies. Interlesional heterogeneity in response to drugs has been extensively studied and its relation to other biologic variables analyzed (Silvestrini et al., 1984). Similarly, much effort has been devoted to in vitro phase II or coresistance studies. In vitro activity of cisplatin (Daidone et al., 1987) or doxorubicin and their analogues has been tested at equivalent clinical concentrations derived from phase I studies on adequate series of previously untreated patients with different tumor types. The outcome of these studies has indicated a similar or higher activity of parent drugs than of the various derivatives and a general overlapping of sensitivity and resistance profiles for drugs of the same family.

Another application of the assay is for the analysis of phenomena of multidrug resistance to unrelated drugs. A study performed on various tumor types showed a significant association in sensitivity or resistance to doxorubicin and vincristine in breast cancers and non-Hodgkin lymphomas but not in testicular tumors (unpublished data).

All these findings, in agreement with experimental and clinical evidence, reinforce the reliability of the in vitro assay and indicate its potential as a valid means for clinically oriented and basic studies.

REFERENCES

Alberts DS, Leigh S, Surwit EA, Serokman R, Moon TE, Salmon SE (1984). Improved survival of patients with relapsing ovarian cancer treated on the basis of drug selection following human tumor clonogenic assay. In Salmon SE, Trent GM (eds): "Human Tumor Cloning," Orlando: Grune and Stratton, p 509.

Daidone MG, Silvestrini R, Sanfilippo O, Zaffaroni N, Varini M, De Lena M (1985). Reliability of an in vitro short-term assay to predict the drug sensitivity of human breast cancer. Cancer 56: 450.

Daidone MG, Silvestrini R, Zaffaroni N, Grignolio E, Landoni F (1987). Absolute and relative activities of platinum-complexes on human tumors as evaluated by an antimetabolic in vitro assay. Invest New Drugs 5: 245.

Del Bino G, Silvestrini R, Costa A, Veneroni S, Giardini R (1986). Morphological and clinical significance of cell kinetics in non-Hodgkin's lymphomas. Basic Appl Histochem 30: 197.

Durie BGM, Vaught L, Soehnlen B, Salmon SE (1982). Sensitivity to interferons and bisantrene in refractory multiple myeloma: comparison between thymidine suppression, myeloma stem cell culture, and clinical results. Annu Meet Am Ass Cancer Res 23: 116.

Goldie JH, Coldman AJ (1979). A mathematical model formulating the drug sensitivity of tumors to their spontaneous mutation rate. Cancer Treat Rep 63: 1727

Meyskens FL, Loescher L, Moon TE, Takasugi B, Salmon SE (1984). Relation of in vitro colony survival to clinical response in a prospective trial of single agent chemotherapy for metastatic melanoma. J Clin Oncol 2: 1223.

Sanfilippo O, Daidone MG, Zaffaroni N, Silvestrini R (1984). Dervelopment of a nucleotide precursor incorporation assay for testing drug sensitivity of human tumors. In Hoffman V, Martz G (eds): "Predictive Drug Testing on Human Tumor Cells," Berlin: Springer Verlag, p 127.

Sanfilippo O, Silvestrini R, Zaffaroni N, Piva L, Pizzocaro G (1986). Appplication of an in vitro antimetabolic assay to human germ cell testicular tumors for the preclinical evaluation of drug sensitivity. Cancer 58: 1441.

Silvestrini R, Daidone MG, Costa A, Sanfilippo O (1985). Cell kinetics and in vitro chemosensitivity as a tool for improved management of patients. Eur J Cancer Clin Oncol 21: 371.

Silvestrini R, Sanfilippo O, Daidione MG (1983). An attempt to use incorporation of radioactive nucleic acid precursors to predict clinical response. In Dendy PP, Hill BT (eds): "Human Tumour Drug Sensitivity Testing In Vitro," London: Academic Press, p 281.

Silvestrini R, Sanfilippo O, Daidone MG, Zaffaroni N (1984). Predictive relevance for clinical outcome of in vitro sensitivity evaluated through antimetabolic assay. In Hoffman V, Martz G (eds): "Predictive Drug Testing on Human Tumor Cells," Berlin: Springer Verlag, p 140.

Tisman G, Herbert V, Edlis H (1973). Determination of therapeutic index of drugs by in vitro sensitivity tests usng human host and tumor cell suspensions. Cancer Chemother Rep 57: 11.

Von Hoff DD (1985). Implications of tumor cell heterogeneity for in vitro drug sensitivity testing. Semin Oncol 12: 327.

Von Hoff DD, Clark GN, Stogdill BJ, Sarosdy MF, et al. (1983). Prospective clinical trial of a human tumor cloning system. Cancer Res 43: 1926

Zaffaroni N, Silvestrini R, Grignolio E, Vaglini M, Motta R (1987). In vitro chemosensitivity testing of human tumors: comparison between an antimetabolic assay and an antiproliferative assay. Proc. 15th Int Congr Chemother, Istanbul (in press).

Supported in part by grants of Italian National Research Council, Specjal Project "Oncology" N. 86.02609.44 and 86.00717.44

Prediction of Response to Cancer Therapy, pages 105–117
© 1988 Alan R. Liss, Inc.

DRUG AND RADIATION SENSITIVITY TESTING OF PRIMARY HUMAN
TUMOR CELLS USING THE ADHESIVE-TUMOR-CELL CULTURE SYSTEM
(ATCCS)

Fraser L. Baker, Gary Spitzer, Jaffer A. Ajani
and William A. Brock

Departments of Hematology and Medical Oncology,
Division of Medicine and the Department of
Experimental Radiotherapy, Division of
Radiotherapy, U.T. M.D. Anderson Hospital and
Tumor Institute, Houston, Texas 77030

INTRODUCTION

Significant clinical responses to chemotherapy can be
achieved, in those patients with tumors sensitive to
therapy. The difficulty is that physicians cannot always
distinguish those patients who might benefit most from
therapy from those unlikely to benefit. The management of
the cancer patient could be positively affected if an in
vitro chemotherapy sensitivity assay able to provide the
oncologist with reliable drug and radiation sensitivity
profiles of the patient's tumor was available.

Several methodologies for sensitivity testing of human
tumors have been published with the greatest number of
reports followed the methodology of in vitro drug
sensitivity testing described by Hamburger and Salmon using
the human tumor stem cell assay (HTSCA) (Hamburger and
Salmon, 1977; Carney et al., 1985; Singletary et al., 1985).
While the HTSCA generated considerable interest in
sensitivity testing for the selection of cancer
chemotherapy, the application of the methodology in a
routine clinical setting was hampered by: technical
difficulties which limited reproducibility, low cloning
efficiency which limited the number of drugs which could be
tested, and low growth efficiency which seriously reduced
the number of patients benefitting from the assay (Selby et
al., 1983).

The main problem with the HTSCA and its modifications has been low colony-forming efficiency. This assay required a high inoculum of 500,000 cells per 35 mm dish to achieve adequate growth. A large amount of tissue is required to evaluate several drugs. The HTSCA is an agar suspension culture method. Suspension cultures are selective and inhibit the growth of anchorage dependent cells (Ben-Zeev and Raz, 1981). Growth in suspension has correlated with tumorigenicity, an accepted marker of malignancy (Shin et al., 1975; Barrett et al., 1979), but this is not absolute (Yates and King, 1982; Marshall et al., 1977; Shields, 1976).

To increase the colony forming efficiency, we developed a monolayer cell culture system that favored growth of anchorage dependent cells called the Adhesive-Tumor-Cell Culture System (ATCCS). The ATCCS is a monolayer cell culture system with a culture surface composed of cell-adhesive matrix (CAM) and culture medium supplemented with serum, hormones and epidermal growth factor (Baker et al., 1986). CAM is a complex mixture of cell-adhesive proteins which also includes both fibronectin and fibrinogen.

The increased growth of primary human tumors cultured on CAM versus tissue culture plastic varied between 1.3 fold and 7 fold (median = 2.3 fold) in nine tests (Table 1). The variability of growth between replicates on CAM was reduced, with the coefficient of variation reduced from 20% on plastic to 5% on CAM in nine tests.

TABLE 1. Characteristics of Growth of Human Tumor Cells on CAM versus Plastic

Tumor	CAM/Plastic	% Coefficient of Variation	
		CAM	Plastic
1	1.2X	5.1	26
2	1.4X	5.5	23
3	1.5X	6.4	40
4	2.1X	6.4	9
5	2.3X	5.7	29
6	3.4X	8.0	28
7	4.4X	3.0	35
8	5.5X	5.6	30
9	7.3X	7.7	25

EGF has a significant effect on the growth rate of human tumor cells in vitro (Singletary et al., 1987). Epidermal growth factor (EGF) increased growth between 0.76 and 20 fold (median = 3.1 fold, n=36) in the ATCCS. The addition of EGF routinely produced colonies containing thousands of cells after 13 days incubation reflecting a cell cycle time of 31 hours.

The colony forming efficiency of the ATCCS was first reported as 0.2% determined from 400 initial primary human tumor cell cultures using Ham's F12 culture medium (Baker et al., 1986) supplemented with hormones, EGF and 10% serum. This colony forming efficiency increased to 2% (400 assays) with a change in culture medium to Eagle's alpha modification of MEM (alphaMEM) and was fairly evenly distributed across tumor types (Baker et al., 1987). This high efficiency permitted a 10 drug sensitivity assay from only 200,000 tumor cells requiring an average biopsy weight of only 0.19 grams.

The morphology of human tumor cells grown in the ATCCS varies from polygonal to fusiform. However, the appearance of cells is influenced by the adhesion to the culture surface (Aplin and Foden, 1982) and by the composition of the culture medium. Papanicolaou staining of day 1 and day 13 coverglass cultures have shown that the cell population grown resembled the starting cell population. The malignant characteristics of the cells grown in the ATCCS have been demonstrated by a variety of methods. Cytoplasmic and nuclear features of malignancy (Figure 1) were found with high frequency. Epithelial cell growth from adenocarcinoma was demonstrated by cytokeratin staining in 6 of 8 cases. Hyperdiploid metaphases (Figure 2) and flow cytometry showed aneuploid tumor cell populations (Figure 3). Human tumor cells harvested from the ATCCS after two weeks were tumorigenic in nude mice in 8 of 12 experiments. These data have confirmed the notion that the ATCCS supports the growth of malignant cells from human cancers.

Considering a colony forming efficiency of 0.1% as reflecting growth, the growth efficiency of the ATCCS was 87% in 400 assays. This high growth efficiency was uniformly distributed across a broad range of tumor types (Table 2) and suggested possible application of the ATCCS in chemotherapy sensitivity testing.

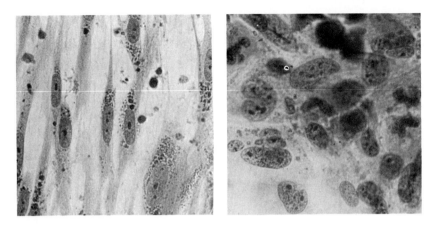

FIGURE 1. Papanicolaou stained, day 13 coverglass cultures
of melanoma (left) and of malignant fibrous histiocytoma
(MFH) (right). The melanoma culture showed elongated cells
with intense melanin pigmentation and the MFH culture showed
dense granular heterochromatin and extreme nuclear
heterogeneity with micronulcei.

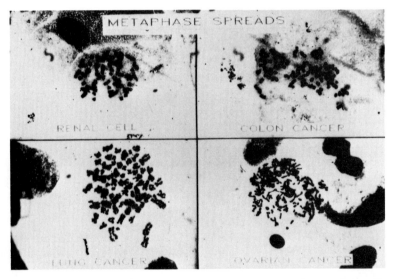

FIGURE 2. Geimsa stained metaphase spreads of renal, colon,
lung and ovarian (clockwise) cancer cells in the ATCCS.
Hyperdiploid metaphases were observed in these cultures.

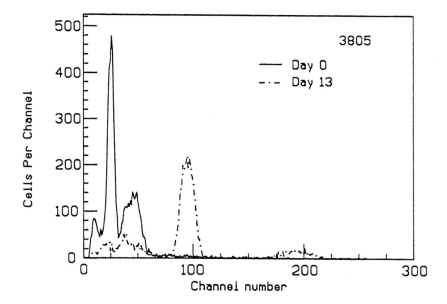

Figure 3. Flow cytometry of starting and cultured ovarian cancer cells. The DNA histogram showed growth of aneuploid cells from a minority of the starting cell population.

TABLE 2. Fraction and percentage of assays with colony forming efficiency > 0.1% by tumor type

Tumor Type	Fraction	Percentage
Breast	40/41	98
Lung	58/65	89
Gynecological	88/111	79
Sarcoma	58/67	87
Melanoma	28/31	90
Gastrointestinal	22/31	71
All tumors	338/398	87

ChemoSensitivity Assay (CSA).

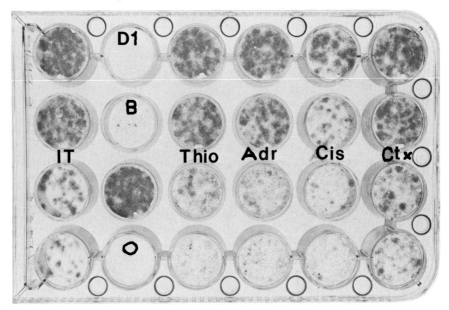

FIGURE 4. Chemosensitivity assay (CSA). An assay for drug
sensitivity based on the ATCCS was developed using 24 well
CAM-Plates (trademark, LifeTrac). The assay determines four
point survival curves for 10 drugs from 200,000 tumor cells
using alphaMEM culture medium. Controls included an inoculum
titration (IT) to determine the 100% value, a culture fixed
after 24 hours incubation to assess the starting cell
population (D1), a thymidine suicide culture (5uC/ml
continuous exposure) to assess the background (non-dividing)
cells (B) and a cell free culture (a blank) (0) for
baseline optical density measurement setting. Test cultures
were set up in the remaining four columns for four drug
survival curves (Thio - thiotepa, Adr - adriamycin, Cis
cisplatin and Ctx - 4 hydroxyperoxycyclophosphamide). The
assay was performed in duplicate. See Ajani et al. 1987 for
further discussion of the CSA. The cultures were incubated for
13 days, then fixed and stained with crystal violet. Cell
staining density (CSD) was quantitated with digital image
analysis. CSD correlated with traditional colony and cell
counts (Figure 5). After one day incubation for cell
attachment, the cultures were washed and drug was added to
the cells. After 6 days of incubation the medium was
exchanged, limiting drug exposure to 5 days. The cultures
were incubated for an additional 7 days.

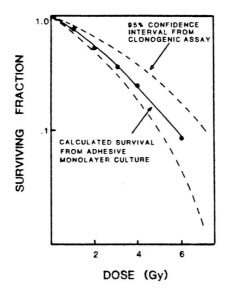

FIGURE 5. Repetitive radiation survival curves were determined for chinese hampster ovary cells (CHO) using colony counts, cell counts, and cell staining density (CSD) values as endpoints and the CSD assay was within the 95 % confidence envelop of conventional assay endpoints.

Drug survival curves show classical log-linear dose response relationships with drugs routinely achieving greater than 1 log quantitation range. A 1:2:4:6 drug dose scale was adopted for all drugs and the end point chosen for the drug was the concentration that achieved 90% inhibition, referred to as IC90 (90 % Inhibitory Concentration). Drug survival curves are shown in Figure 6.

The in vitro drug dosages used in the CSA were normalized to their responsiveness in the chemosensitivity assay. For example, the dosages were adjusted such that a 15 % IC90 response rate was achieved at the second dilution of the drug. These concentrations are approximately the same range as for inhibition of granulocyte/macrophage colony-forming cells for myelosuppressive drugs and are higher for non-myelosuppresive drugs (Table 3) (Ajani et al., 1986). The similarity of average IC90 values for human tumors and granulocyte/macrophage colony-forming cells (GM-CFC) for

myelosuppressive drugs suggest that the GM-CFC could be a
good method for establishing in vitro dose for
myelosuppressive drugs (Fan et al., 1987).

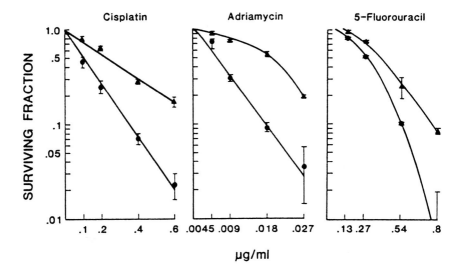

FIGURE 6. Typical cisplatin, adriamycin and fluorouracil
drug survival curves for two tumors of different
sensitivity. The end point of the CSA is the drug
concentration that inhibited 90 % of growth (IC90).

TABLE 3. Comparison of average drug IC90 values
for human tumors and GM-CFC.

Drug	GM-CFC IC90	Human Tumor IC90	GM-CFC/Tumor IC90 ratio
Adriamycin	0.0078	0.0065	1.20
BCNU	4.0	2.99	1.34
Bleomycin	2.5	0.022	113
Cisplatin	0.92	0.29	3.17
Fluorouracil	0.76	0.31	2.45
Mitomycin	0.015	0.010	1.50
Vincristine	0.0022	0.0014	1.57
Etoposide	0.113	0.132	0.86

In vitro drug sensitivity was determined by comparing the drug's IC90 value to the distribution of accumulated responses for that drug and calling sensitivity when the IC90 value was within the 15th percentile. The distribution of cisplatin responses shown in Figure 7 illustrates the method used to determine in vitro drug sensitivity. Retrospective clinical correlations of the CSA have been achieved considering the in vitro cutoff suggested above and a clinical response defined as a partial or complete response. A true positive correlation rate of 76 % and a true negative correlation rate of 96 % was observed (Table 4) (Ajani et al., 1987).

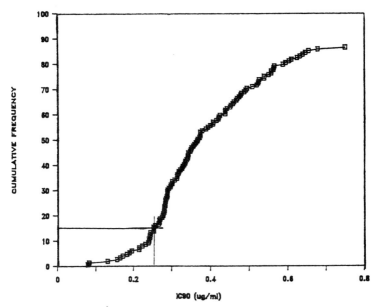

FIGURE 7. Cumulative frequency distribution of 148 human. tumor IC90 responses to cisplatin, showing the 15th percentile cut offused to define in vitro sensitivity.

TABLE 4. In vivo/in vitro clinical correlations from 71 trials			
S/S*	R/S*	R/S*	R/R*
13/17	4/17	3/54	51/54

* S = sensitive, R = resistant

Radiation Sensitivity Assay (RSA).

Radiation effect on cell growth resulted in classical survival curves in the ATCCS (Figure 8). Since the radiation sensitivity assay evaluates only one modality, a more rigorous assay was established in which an 8 point survival curve over the range of 0.75 Gy to 5 Gy was generated at four inocula in duplicate. This assay required only 200,000 tumor cells and provided enough data to restrict the analysis to cultures with linear inoculum titrations (Brock et al., 1987). The end point for measuring in vitro radiation sensitivity was survival fraction at 2 Gray of radiation after Fertil and Malaise (1981). The distribution of this end point by tumor type is in agreement with data published for human cell lines (Figure 9) (Fertil and Malaise, 1985).

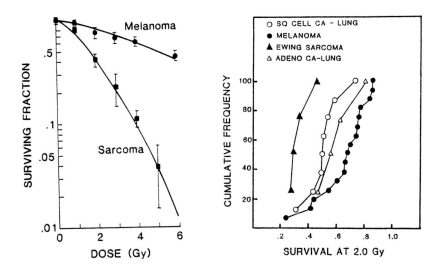

FIGURE 8 (left). Typical radiation survival curves for two tumors of different sensitivity. The end point of the RSA is the survival fraction at 2 Gray of radiation.

FIGURE 9 (right). Distribution of sensitivity of tumors of different histologies to ionizing raditaion. The known sensitive tumor histologies were most sensitive in vitro.

SUMMARY

In summary, the ATCCS is an efficient culture system which grows clonogenic cells from greater than 80 % of human cancers.

The ATCCS supports the growth of malignant cells from human cancers.

The ATCCS shows classical drug and radiation survival curves which routinely achieve over 1 log of kill.

The ATCCS has high CFE and permits sensitivity testing from small samples.

Clinical correlations for the chemosensitivity assay were satisfactory.

Radiosensitivity in vitro correlates with tumor histology.

ACKNOWLEDGEMENT
We are grateful to Dr. Robert Ozols for his review of this work and his presentation of this manuscript. This work was supported by a grant from LifeTrac, Irvine, California.

REFERENCES

Ajani J, Blaauw AA, Spitzer G, Baker FL, Tomasovic B, Umbach G, Thielvoldt D, Zander AR, Dicke KA. Differential cytotoxic activity of chemotherapy agents on colony-forming cells from human tumors and normal bone marrow in vitro. Exp Hematol 13:95-100, 1986.

Ajani JA, Baker FL, Spitzer G, Kelly A, Brock WA, Tomasovic B, Singletary SE, Mcmurtrey M, Plager C. Comparison between clinical response and in vitro drug sensitivity of primary human tumors in the adhesive-tumor-cell culture system. J Clin Oncol, In Press, 1987.

Aplin JD, Foden LJ. A cell spreading factor abundant in human placenta contains fibronectin and fibrinogen. J Cell Sci 58:287-302, 1982.

Baker FL, Spitzer G, Ajani JA, Brock WA, Lukeman J, Pathak S, Tomasovic B, Thielvoldt D, Williams M, Vines C, Tofilon P. Drug and radiation sensitivity measurements of successful primary monolayer culturing of human tumor cells using cell-adhesive matrix and supplemented culture medium. Cancer Res 46:1263-1274, 1986.

Baker FL, Ajani JA, Spitzer G, Tomasovic B, Williams M, Finders M, Trillet V, Brock WA. High colony-forming efficiency of primary human tumor cells cultured in the adhesive-tumor-cell culture system: improvements with medium and serum alterations. Submitted, 1987.

Barrett JC, Crawford BD, Mixter LO, Schechtman IM, Ts'o POP, Pollack R. Correlation of in vitro growth properties and tumorigenicity of syrian hamster cell lines. Cancer Res 39:1504-1510, 1979.

Ben-Zeev A, Raz A. Multinucleation and inhibition of cytokinesis in suspended cells: reversal upon reattachment to a substrate. Cell 26:107-115, 1981.

Brock WA, Baker FL, Peters LJ, Spitzer G, Bock S, Williams M. Radiosensitivity of human tumor cells in culture. Proc Natl Acad Sc, in press, 1987.

Carney DN, Winkler CF. In vitro assays of chemotherapeutic sensitivity. Devita VT. (Ed.) Important Advances in Oncology 1985. pgs. 78-103, Philadelphia, Pennsylvania, USA, 1985.

Fan DF, Ajani JA, Baker FL, Tomasovic B, Brock WA, Spitzer G. Comparison of antitumor activity of standard and investigational drugs at equivalent granulocyte-macrophage colony forming cell inhibitory concentrations in the adhesive-tumor-cell culture system: An in vitro method of screening new drugs. Eur J Cancer Clin Oncol, In Press, 1987.

Fertil B, Malaise EP. Inherent cellular radiosensitivity as a basic concept for human tumor radiotherapy. Int J Radiat Oncol Biol Phys 7:621-629, 1981.

Fertil B, Malaise EP. Intrinsic radiosensitivity of human cell lines is correlated with radioresponsiveness of human tumors: analysis of 101 published survival curves. Int J Rad Oncol Biol Phys 11: 1699-1707, 1985.

Hamburger AM, Salmon SE. Primary bioassay of human tumor
stem cells. Science 197:461-463, 1977.

Marshall CJ, Franks IM, Carbonell AW. Markers of neoplastic
transformation in epithelial cell lines derived from
human carcinomas. J Natl Cancer Inst 58:1743-1747, 1977.

Selby P, Buick RN, Tannock I. A critical appraisal of the
"human tumor stem-cell assay". New Engl J Med 308:129-134,
1983.

Shields R. Transformation and tumorigenicity. Nature
262:348-350, 1976.

Shin S, Freedman VH, Risser R, Pollack R. Tumorigenicity of
virus-transformed cells in nude mice is correlated
specifically with anchorage independent growth in vitro.
Proc Nat Acad Sc 72:4435-4439, 1975.

Singletary SE, Umbach GE, Spitzer G, Drewinko B, Tomasovic
B, Ajani J, Hug V, Blumenschein G. The human tumor stem
cell assay revisited. Int J Cell Clon 3:116-128, 1985.

Singletary SE, Baker FL, Spitzer G, Tucker SL, Tomasovic B,
Brock WA, Ajani JA, Kelly AM. Biological effect of
epidermal growth factor on the in vitro growth of human
tumors. Cancer Res 47:403-406, 1987.

Yates J, King RJB. Lack of correlation between transformed
characteristics in culture and tumorigenicity of mouse
mammary tumor cells. Eur J Cancer Clin Oncol 18:399-404,
1982.

Prediction of Response to Cancer Therapy, pages 119–137
© 1988 Alan R. Liss, Inc.

PREDICTIVE TESTS FOR CANCER CHEMOTHERAPY AND THE PROBLEM
OF TUMOR CELL HETEROGENEITY

Youcef M. Rustum
Harry K. Slocum
Department of Experimental Therapeutics,
Grace Cancer Drug Center, Roswell Park
Memorial Institute, 666 Elm Street,
Buffalo, NY 14263

INTRODUCTION AND RESULTS

During the last several years investigations have
been directed toward the development of means for the
identification of determinants of drug action and their
relevance to prediction of response. Many of these
approaches concentrated primarily on the development of
in vitro assay using a variety of biochemical, pharmaco-
logical, biological and molecular techniques. Although
some success has been achieved utilizing leukemia cells,
progress in the area of solid tumor is at their infancy.
This probably is due in part to the model system when
leukemia cells are present in a single suspension, highly
viable and multiple sample may be obtained. In contrast, in solid tumors the presence of many cell types
with different types and degrees of viability, accom-
panied with limited sample sizes and accessibility and
the need for tumor tissue disaggregation hindered the
progress in the development of quantitation in vitro predictive assays for drug action and response.

In recent years predictive assays based on in vitro
biochemical characterization of tumor cells have been
developed and utilized for prediction of response of
acute leukemia patients to treatment with arabinosylcytosine (araC) (Rustum and Preisler, 1979; Preisler, Rustum
and Priore, 1985). In solid tumors, efforts in this
laboratory have been concentrating on the development of

methods for tumor tissue disaggregation, characterization
so that maximum yield and viability may be obtained. In
addition, development of in vitro growth assays for
assessing tumor cell heterogeneity in terms of growth and
response are also underway.

The human tumor colony formation assay (HTCFA) was
conceptually described and popularized by Hamburger and
Salmon and coworkers about 1980 (Hamburger et al, 1978;
Salmon, 1980) as a method of determining the chemosensitivity of human tumors on an individual patient
basis. A number of difficulties have prevented the HTCFA
from realizing its full potential (editorial, 1982), and
among these are the presence of cell aggregates in cell
suspensions, and insufficient colony formation in many
specimens. Two of the approaches which have been employed to reduce the first problem are likely to increase
the second as outlined below:

Why not eliminate aggregates by better disaggregation, or
by filtration?

It is virtually impossible to produce absolutely
monodisperse cell suspensions directly from surgical
samples of human carcinomas (Mattern and Volm, 1982;
Agrez et al, 1982; Slocum et al, 1984; Slocum et al,
1985), and in our experience it is also not desirable.
At least in some samples most of the colonies are formed
from aggregates directly (Agrez et al, 1982; Slocum et
al, 1984; Slocum et al, 1985), or their growth is supported by the presence of aggregates indirectly (Slocum
et al, 1984; Slocum et al, 1985). In principle one might
expect that cells involved in aggregates might possess
growth advantages over those removed from their neigh-
bors, as discussed above in considering the collagen-gel
growth system of Freeman and Hoffman (Freeman and
Hoffman, 1986), and as has been suggested by Yang et al
(Yang et al, 1980) and Miller et al (Miller et al, 1985)
in design of a similar collagen culture system for tumor
tissues (Slocum et al, 1985). In fact for human breast
tissue, the optimal method for producing primary cultures
involves the disaggregation of tissue only to the level
of cell clusters, which contain the cell population of
interest (Stampfer et al, 1980; Smith et al, 1981).
Thus, eliminating aggregates may seriously reduce the
growth potential of the culture, and this is obviously a

counterproductive approach in light of poor colony forming capacity in many samples.

Why not subtract aggregate counts from final colony counts?

This approach has been taken for larger aggregates ("colony" sized) at the time of plating. Again this reduces the useful growth potential of the culture by eliminating the growth of large aggregates from inclusion in the assay. If a laboratory adopts a rule of discarding the test if more than 15 large aggregates appear on control plates at time zero, this further increases the number of samples for which the test is unsuitable. This approach also takes no account of sub-colony sized aggregates (e.g. 2-30 cells), which are more numerous in most suspensions. Interpretation of colony counts is difficult when it is unknown whether a 32-cell colony arose from a 10-cell aggregate or a single cell. A more detailed discussion of the consequences of inadequately dealing with aggregates during the analysis of colony formation assays is presented by Rockwell (Rockwell, 1985).

How can high resolution image analysis address these problems?

Image analysis has been applied to the evaluation of colony formation assays to bring a measure of automation to a labor-intensive technique (Salmon, 1980; Kahn et al, 1986; Herman et al, 1983; Kallman, 1984), but has not been designed to deal with the problems discussed above. The approach we have designed, and are implementing employs optics of sufficient resolution to follow growth at the individual colony level. This is not a new concept; (Kallman, 1984; Rauthe et al, 1981) have previously reported the use of time lapse cinematography to monitor growth of individual colonies. Unfortunately these photographic approaches are not amenable to precise quantitation in a totally automated way, and therefore of limited utility. The electronic time lapse approach is automatable, and will allow quantitation of growth through time of thousands of cells in each culture simultaneously. This makes available the maximum information a colony formation assay can render, in that all growth, whether from single cells or aggregates, can be precisely

quantitated. Thus, the growth of aggregates can contribute to the useful signal in the assay, and serve to
increase rather than decrease the number of samples for
which growth can be measured.

In addition to addressing difficulties encountered
with the HTCFA for prediction of clinical chemosensitivity, the design of the assay makes it useful for
obtaining maximum information from colony formation by
cells derived from clinical specimens, human tumor xenografts, or established cell lines. Since the information
obtained pertains to the individual colony, direct observation of cellular heterogeneity in response to pro-
liferation-modifying agents is possible. At present, up
to 1800 growth events can be followed simultaneously in
each culture, providing previously unobtainable data to
which to fit mathematical models of proliferation and
effects of drugs and drug sensitivity on proliferation.
Since the design allows for correlative microscopy
studies on individual colonies, previously untestable
hypotheses relating specific cellular parameters to
proliferation should become testable.

Biochemical and molecular techniques for defining the
basis for drug responsiveness often require purified, or
at least subpopulation-enriched, suspensions. We have
employed centrifugal elutriation (Slocum et al, 1985;
Keng et al, 1981), density gradient centrifugation
(Kopper et al, 1982), and flow cytometeric cell sorting
to achieve subpopulation enrichment from cell suspensions
derived from human surgical specimens. Flow cell sorting
of cells directly from disaggregated human solid tumors
is a new achievement, and should make available nearly
pure subpopulations for assays requiring relatively small
numbers of cells, such as the colony formation assay
discussed above. Centrifugal elutriation has been useful
for enriching for aneuploid populations (Slocum et al,
1985; Keng et al, 1981), and should benefit from new cell
adhesive protein derivatives (Picciano and Benedict,
1986) and techniques for encouraging cells to adhere to
substrates (Balcavage et al, 1987), in that recovery and
subsequent culture of elutriated cells may be markedly
improved. Density gradient centrifugation has been
useful for enriching for tumor cells (Keng et al, 1981),
but has suffered from poor cell recoveries due to aggre-

gation of cells in fractions. Implantation of aggregated fractions under the renal capsule of nude mice or immune suppressed mice (Fingert et al, 1984) is another approach which may turn a previous disadvantage (cell aggregation) into an advantage. Thus techniques recently developed offer new advantages to approaches which previously have been only partly successful.

In Vitro Assay for Prediction of Response of Patients with Acute Nonlymphocytic Leukemia.

While current chemotherapeutic regimens induce a high proportion of remissions in previously untreated patients with acute myelocytic leukemia, fewer than 50% of patients has a remission which lasts for more than three years (Keating et al, 1985; Capizzi et al, 1985; Lazarus et al, 1981; Rustum and Preisler, 1979). The majority of patients die within two years of diagnosis as a result of relapsed disease or of having never entered remission initially. Chemotherapeutic regimens currently in use have been empirically derived without knowing the specific factors which play a role in determining an individual patient's responsiveness to chemotherapy. It is clear that remission induction and long-term survival are due to the interaction of many factors including the biological characteristics of the host and the sensitivity of the leukemic cells to the chemotherapeutic agents administered. The administration of a drug to a patient whose leukemic cells are resistant results in host toxicity without therapeutic benefit.

Recent advances in the treatment of ANLL patients (with high dose araC alone and in combination with other agents), especially high risk and relapsed patients, suggested that "resistance" to conventional doses of araC may be circumvented at higher peak plasma concentrations of araC. These clinical results suggest that the transport of araC may be the rate limiting step. However, additional factors such as araCTP formation, retention and incorporation into DNA may play an important role in circumvention of resistance to araC (Rustum, 1978; Rustum et al, 1982; Iacoboni et al, 1986; Plunkett et al, 1985; Kufe et al, 1982; Momparler et al, 1986; Kufe et al, 1985; Major et al, 1982).

In vitro and in vivo studies with araC in leukemia cells obtained from previously untreated ANLL patients demonstrated that: 1) metabolism of araC is efficient at low doses, (Riva et al, 1985; Rustum and Preisler, 1987; Riva and Rustum, 1985) in the majority of cases tested; 2) in vitro araCTP retention at 4 hr predicted for duration of complete response but not for induction of CR; 3) intensive consolidation (P970701) with higher doses of araC decreased the prognostic value of araCTP retention (Chart 1); and 4) both in vitro and in vivo results demonstrated the existence of a subgroup of ANLL patients with low level or deficiency in CdR kinase. In

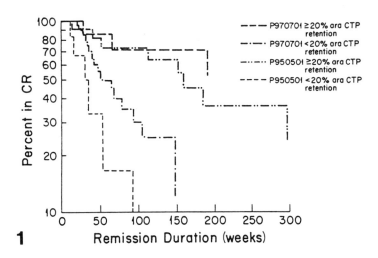

1 Remission Duration (weeks)

relapsed ANLL patients (Chart 2): 1)similar degrees of heterogeneity in araCTP formation and retention were

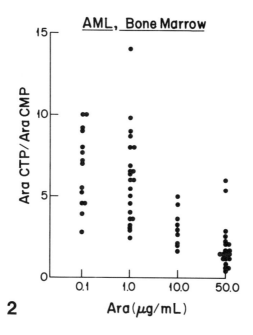

2

observed; 2) in a majority of cases higher doses are required for optimization of the intracellular araCTP pools (Chart 3); 3) a lack of relationship between plasma araC and cellular araCTP was demonstrated; 4) in relapsed and high risk patients araC doses higher than 1.0 g/m^2 did not appear to have an additional effect on araCTP accumulation; 5) in high risk patients, similar response rates were achieved in patients treated with 2 and 3 gm/m^2 and 6) significant differences in in vivo araCTP retention 11 hr following the administration of 3g/m^2 araC were demonstrated.

Studies by Plunkett and his coworkers (Iacoboni et al, 1986; Plunkett et al, 1985) have demonstrated also the importance of cellular pharmacology of araC, namely, araCTP pools and retention in relapsed ANLL patients. Data generated, therefore, in our laboratory demonstrated

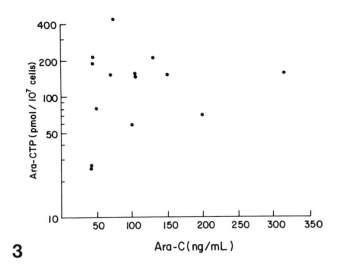

3

a large degree of heterogeneity in the cellular pharmacology of araC of patients receiving high dose araC
treatments ($3g/m^2/12$ hr). Furthermore, the peak plasma
concentration of araC was always greater than 100μM, a
concentration more than sufficient for saturation of
araCTP formation (Chart 4). In fact, 10μM araC is sufficient to saturate dCMP-kinase, the enzyme responsible for
conversion of araCMP to araCDP. Thus, these pharmaco-
logical data taken together with the clinical experience
with $3g/m^2/$araC clearly demonstrate that we are over
treating and perhaps under these conditions, the selectivity of araC against tumor cells is completely lost.
In fact our results in mice bearing tumors have demonstrated that when araCTP ratios in tumor and normal bone
marrow cells approach unity, toxicity predominates.

Since we have demonstrated a strong relationship
between the in vitro araCTP retention, and duration of
complete response and also that intensive consolidation
therapy has reduced the prognostic importance of these
determinants, studies are underway to evaluate the biochemical basis for this phenomenon and to propose approaches to overcome this specific type of pharmaco-

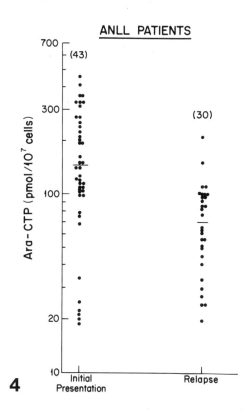

logical limitation. In this reguard, the use of a newly
synthesized araC prodrug, araC-PTBA (Hong et al, 1986;
Hong et al, 1987; Berdel et al, 1987), the utilization of
liposome encapsulated araC (Mayhew et al, 1983; Fllens et
al, 1982; Rustum et al, 1981; Mayhew et al, 1979),
evaluation of deoxycytidine monophosphate deaminase inhibitor, deoxytetrahydrourridine (Fridland et al, 1986;
Verhoef and Fridland, 1986; Boothman et al, 1985; Mekras
et al, 1983, Greer and Mekras, 1983; Fridland et al,
1986; Mekras et al, 1984) and deoxycytidine deaminase

inhibitor, tetrahydrouridine (Briggle, 1986; Perez et al, 1984; Riccardi et al, 1982; Ho et al, 1980; Kreis et al, 1977; Kreis et al, 1977; Kreis et al, 1977; Kreis et al., 1987; Kreis et al, 1977), are a few examples of agents that would be evaluated to overcome resistance due to rapid degradation of cellular araCTP. The significance of the in vitro studies with these agents is that araCTP formation, retention, incorporation into DNA and the extent of inhibition and duration of dThyd incorporation onto DNA can be evaluated in cells of all patients. Thus, the selective advantage of these agents and approaches in a specific patient population subtype can be fully documented.

In summary, studies conducted to date demonstrated that indeed in vitro biochemical assays are useful techniques for prediction of patient outcome to therapy. This assay is rapidly requiring less than 24 h and additional applications may be to define the dose of schedule of drug treatment for optimal therapeutic selectivity.

Development of In Vitro Growth Assays for Prediction of Response in Solid Tumors.

a. Cell Yield from Solid Tumor Tissue

Two approaches have been taken to improve the effective yields of cells from solid tumors: 1) a direct approach of attempting to fractionate the enzyme mixture used in the disaggregation procedure to eliminate possible cytodestructive activities and retain disaggregation activity, 2) an indirect approach of implementing an in vitro tissue culture system for solid tumor tissues, to allow the cells a period of recovery from removal in vivo, and expand the tumor material available from individual patients.

1) Initial attempts to fractionate the enzyme mixture we have found most useful for disaggregating most types of human tumors have included the classical protein fractionation methods of ammonium sulfate precipitation, gel filtration, and ion-exchange chromatography. No fraction so obtained has demonstrated activity which is superior or even equal to the activity of the whole mixture. It

seems likely that multiple enzyme activities are required simultaneously to achieve the disaggregation effect, and their copurification may be unlikely by any simple approach. No major effort to pursue this line of improvement is currently planned.

2) A method has recently been described by Freeman and Hoffman (Freeman and Hoffman, 1986) for the culture of human tumor tissue pieces on sponges derived from collagen gel. Our early experience with this culture system appears promising; a summary appears in Table 1. Six 1 mm^2 pieces of tumor tissue were planted on a 1 cm^2 gel pad. In the table: 1 = growth noted as expansion of all tumor pieces, 2 = growth resulting in the borders of all pieces coming into contact, 3 = growth

Table 1

Type of Tumor	Total	Number of Tumors Contaminated	Growing	No Growth	Tumor Growth 1	2	3	Gel Erosion +	-
Sarcoma	32	3	17	12	11	5	1	7	22
Ovarian	16	4	8	4	5	2	1	4	8
Colon	14	6	8		3	4	1	4	4
Breast	18	2	12	4	6	4	2	10	6
Lung	15	2	12	1	6	4	2	6	7
Gastric	5	0	5	0	1	4	0	3	2
Prostate	3	0	3	0	1	2	0	1	3
Melanoma	4	1	2	1	2	0	0	0	3
Kidney	2	1	0	1	0	0	0	0	1
Other	6	1	5	1	1	2	1	2	4
TOTAL	115	19	72	24	37	27	8	37	59

to confluent mass. While a simple approach to assessing growth has been taken initially, a more quantitative approach employing image analysis is under development. If growth in category 2 or 3 only are considered a success, the technique was successful in an encouraging fraction of cases (30%). We expect that the autoradiographic approach of Freeman and Hoffman (Freeman and Hoffman, 1986) will verify a success ratio between 30 and

63%. A sample of small cell lung carcinoma which failed to grow in the colony formation assay or on an extra-cellular matrix-like substrate (Matrigel) directly from surgery, grew in both systems after 3 weeks culture on the collagen matrix. This has also become a cell line on standard plastic culture vessels (Slocum et al, manu-script in preparation).

b. Use of Image Analysis System

We have designed a high resolution image analysis (HRIA) approach which follows individual colony formation events through time, and allows certain correlative microscopic studies to characterize the cells comprising colonies with known growth rates. Basically the system works by making electronic time lapse photographs of the agar culture, identifying and measuring each feature through time. Two major advantages acrue from this approach: 1) the image analyzer does not have to be taught to differentiate between true colonies and inert objects in the culture, as the quantitation is based on growth through time rather than simply on size at any given point in time, and 2) the growth of clusters of cells can be quantitated through time, thus obviating the need to "subtract" time zero counts and ignore the growth potential of cells involved in aggregates.

Initially, glass marker beads were utilized to demonstrate that individual objects in the agar could be correctly identified repeatedly, and that growth events did not appear artifactually. Details of the physical requirements of the culture and analysis system appear in other reports as well as a description of the pertinent software (Slocum et al, 1987a,b).

Cell lines were plated and followed for basic proliferation pattern through time, to lay the groundwork for assessment of drug effect an example of such experiment appears below.

A human colon carcinoma cell line, COLO 205 (Semple and et al., 1978), was plated in the agarose system and binary images stored for 16 fields of view through time. Subsequently, the binary records were recalled from the computer, measured, matched, and the area of each colony

through time recorded. Chart 5 represents a growth curve
for 100 representative colonies and demonstrates the
heterogeneity in growth rates of individual events on the
plate. The doubling times were calculated as volume
doubling times from the rate of increasing area under the
assumption that the colonies grow as oblate spheroids, as
has been indicated by Meyskens group (Meyskens et al,
1984; Thomson et al, 1984) for several other cell lines

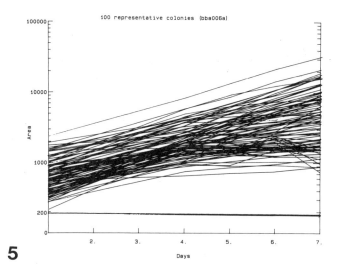

5

and human melanoma primary cultures. While we have only
preliminary verification of this for COLO 205 cells, we
still use it as a first approximation until confirmatory
studies are accomplished. Viability was determined
through use of a metabolizable tetrazolium dye, MTT
(Klebe et al, 1984). 72% of objects followed showed
viability on day 8. The median doubling time for viable
colonies was 29 hours (Interquartile range = 22.3 - 43.8
hours). the capability of following growth events on an
individual colony basis with correlation to metabolic
capability should be a valuable tool to determine
cellular heterogeneity of growth rate and response to
antiproliferative agents.

REFERENCES

Agrez, MV, Kovach JS, Lieber MM (1982). Cell Aggregates in the Soft Agar "human tumour stem-cell assay." Br J Cancer 46:880-887, p. 65,66.

Balcavage WX, Jones M, Balcavage E (1987). Rapid Cell Plating with a Cell Centrifuge. American Biotechnology Laboratory.

Berdel W, Danhauser S, Schick H, Fromm, M, Fink U, Hons C-I, Reichert A and Rastetter J (1987). Proc Am Assoc Cancer Pes 28 (Abst. No. 1203).

Boothman DA, Prissle TV, Greer S (1985). Metabolic Channeling of 5-fluoro-2'-deoxycytidine Utilizing Inhibitors of its Deamination in Cell Culture. Mol Pharmacol 27(5):584-594.

Briggle (1986) T. The Biochemical Basis for the Selective Antitumor Activity of 5-Fluoro-2'-Deoxycytidine when Coadministered wth Tetrahydrouridine. Diss Abstr Int B 47(3):1032.

Capizzi RL, Powell BL, Cooper MR, Cruz MR, Lyerly S, Posenbaum D, Muss H, Richards F, White D and Jackson D (1987). Sequential High-Dose AraC and Asparaginase in the Therapy of Previously Treated and Untreated Patients with Acute Leukemia. Proc Am Soc Clin Oncol 6:A645.

editorial (1982). Clonogenic Assays for the Chemotherapeutic Sensitivity of Human Tumours. Lancet 1(part 2):780-781.

Ellens H, Rustum Y, Mayhew E, Ledesma E (1982). Distribution and Metabolism of Liposome-encapsulated AraC. J Pharmacol Expt Therapeutics 222:324-330.

Fingert HJ, Treiman A, Pardee AB (1984). Transplantation of Human or Rodent Tumors into Cyclosporine-treated Mice: A Feasible Model for Studies of Tumor Biology and Chemotherapy. Proc Acad Sci USA 81:7927-7931.

Freeman AE, Hoffman RM (1986). In Vivo-like Growth of Human Tumors In Vitro. Proc Natl Acad Sci 83:2604-2698.

Fridland A, Verhoef V, Mirro J., Jr, Dahl GV (1986). Effects of the Deaminase Inhibitor 2'-Deoxytetrahydrouridine (DTHU) on AraC Metabolism in Leukemic and Normal Human Marrow Leukocytes. Proc Am Assoc Cancer Res 27:372.

Fridland A, Verhoef V, Mirro J Jr, Dahl GV (1986). Effects of the Deaminase Inhibitor 2'-Deoxytetrahydrouridine on Cytosine Arabinoside Metabolism in Leukemic and Normal Human Marrow Leukocytes. UICC, 14th International Cancer Congress, Budapest, Hungary, August 21-27.

Gale RP (1979). Advances in the Treatment of Acute Myelogeneous Leukemia. New England J Med 300:1189-1199.

Greer S, Mekras J (1983). Marked Enhancement of the Cytotoxicity of 5-Fluorodeoxyuridine by Deoxytetrahydrouridine, a Nontoxic Analog that Affects Deoxyuridylate Levels. Fed Proc 42(4):768, 1983.

Hamburger AW, Salmon SE, Kim MB, Trent JM, Soehnlein BJ, Alberts DC, Schmidt HJ (1978). Direct Cloning of Human Ovarian Carcinoma Cells in Agar. Cancer Res 38:3438-3444.

Herman CJ, Pelgrim OE, Kirkels WJ, Verheijen R (1983). In Use Evaluation of the Omnicon Automated Tumor Colony Counter. Cytometry 3:439-442.

Ho DHW, Carter CJ, Brown NS, Hester J, McCredie K, Benjamin RS, Freireich EJ and Bodey GP (1980). Effects of Tetrahydrouridine on the Uptake and Metabolism of 1-β-D-Arabinofuranosylcytosine in Human Normal and Leukemic Cells. Cancer Res 40:2411-2446.

Hong C, Buchheit D, Kiristis A, Nechaev A, West CR, Bernacki RJ and Hui SW (1987). AraC-thioether-phospholipid Conjugate. Proc Am Assoc Cancer Res 28 (Abst. No. 1203).

Hong C, Kirisits AJ, Bucheit DJ, Nechaev A and West CR (1986). 1-β-D-Arabinofuranosylcytosine-phospholipid Conjugates as Prodrug of AraC. Cancer Drug Delivery 3:101.

Iacoboni SJ, Plunkett W, Kantarjian HM, Ester F, Keatings MJ, McCredie KB and Freireich EJ (1986). High-Dose AraC Treatment and Cellular Pharmacology of Chronic Myelogenous Leukemia Blast Crisis. J Clin Oncol 4:1079-1088.

Kahn E., Benard J, Di Paola R (1986). The Use of An Image Analyser in Human Tumor Clonogenic Assays. Cytometry 7:313-317.

Kallman RF (1984). Automated autoradiographic analysis of tumor cell colonies in vitro. In Eisert WG, Mendelsohn ML (eds): "Biological Dosimetry", Berlin Heidelberg: Springer-Verlag, pp 254-263.

Keating MJ, Estey W, Plunkett W, Iacoboni S, Walters R, Kantarjian H, Andersson B, Beran M, McCredie KB and Freireich EJ (1985). Evolution of Clinical Studies with High Dose Cytosine Arabinoside at the M.D. Anderson Hospital. Seminars in Oncol 12(2)Supp. 3:98-104.

Keng PC, Wheeler FT, Siemann DW, Lord EM (1981). Direct Synchronization of Cells from Solid Tumors by Centrifugal elutriation. Exp Cell Res 134:15-22.

Kopper L, Casillo S, Rustum Y, Slocum HK, Frankfurt O, Takita H (1982). Separation and Characterization of Human Tumor Cells on a Discontinuous Percoll Gradient. Proc Am Assoc Cancer Pes 23:30 (Abst. No. 114).

Kreis W, Chan K, Budman DP, Shulman P, Allen S, Weiselberg L, Henderson V, Freeman J, Deere M and Vincisuerra V (1986). Effect of Tetrahydrouridine (THU) on AraC Pharmacokinetics and Toxicity when Both Drugs are Given by continuous Infusion over 3 hrs. Proc Assoc Cancer Pes 27:165.

Kreis W, Hession C, Soricelli A, Scully K (1977). Combination of THU and AraC in Mouse Tumor. Cancer Treat Pepts 61:1355-1364.

Kreis W, Woodcock TM, Gordon CS, Drakoff IH (1977). Tetrahydrouridine: Physiologic Disposition and Fffect upon Deamination of Cytosine Arabinoside in Man. Cancer Treat Repts 61:1347-1353.

Kreis W., Woodcock TM, Gordon CS, Drakoff IH (1977). THU: PHysiologic Disposition and Effect Upon Deamination of Cytosine Arabinoside. Cancer Treat Pepts 61:1347-1353.

Kufe DW, Major PP, Fgan M, Beardsley P (1982). Correlation of cytotoxicity with Incorporatio of AraC into DNA. J biol Chem 31:2937-2940.

Kufe SW, Sprigs DP (1985). Biochemical and Cellular Pharmacology of AraC. Seminars in Oncol 12(2)Supp. 3:34-48.

Lazarus H, Herzig G, Herzig P, Phillips GL, Roessmann U, and Fishman DJ (1981). Central Nervous System Toxicity of High Dose AraC. Cancer 48:2577-2582.

Major P, Fgan F, Beardsley G, Minden M, Kufe D (1982). Lethality of Human Myeloblasts Correlates with the Incorporation of AraC into DNA. Proc Natl Acad Sci 78:3253-3259.

Mattern J, Volm M. (1982). Clinical Relevance of Predictive Tests for Cancer Chemotherapy. Canc Treat
Pev 9:267-298.

Mayhew E, Pustum Y, Szoka F and Papahadjopoulos D
(1979). Role ofCholesterol in Enhancing the
Antitumor Activity of AraC in Liposomes. Cancer
Treat Report 63:1923-1928.

Mayhew E, Rustum Y, Vail W (1983). Effects of Liposome
Entrapped Chemotherapeutic Agents on Mouse Primary
and Metastatic Tumors. Biol of Cell 47:81-86.

Mekras J and Greer S (1983). Use of 5-Fluorodeoxy-
cytidine and Tetrahydrouridine to Exploit High Levels
of Deoxycytidylate Deaminase in Tumors: Target
Directed Conversion of a Nontoxic Analog to a Toxic
Antimetabolite. Fed Proc 42(3):360.

Mekras JA, Boothman DA, Perez LM, Greer S (1984). Use of
5-Fluorodeoxycytidine and Tetrahydrouridine to
Exploit High Levels of Deoxycytidylate Deaminase in
Tumors to Achieve DNA- and Target-Directed
Therapies. Cancer Res 44(6):2551-2560.

Mekras JA, Boothman DA, Perez LAM, Greer S (1984). Use
of 5-Fluorodeoxycytidine and Tetrahydrouridine to
Exploit High Levels of Deoxycytidylate Deaminase in
Tumors to Achieve DNA Directed and Target Directed
Therapies. Cancer Res 44(6)2551-2560.

Meyskens FL, Jr, Thomson SP, Moon TE (1984). Quantita-
tion of the Number of Cells Within Tumor Colonies in
Semisolid Medium and Their Growth as Oblate
Spheroids. Cancer Res 44:271-277.

Miller BE, Miller FP, Heppner GH (1985). Factors Affecting Growth and Drug Sensitivity of Mouse Mammary
Tumor Lines in Collagen Gel Cultures. Cancer Res
45:4200-4205.

Momparler PL, Onetto N, Momparler LF, Gyser M, Leclerc JM
and Rivard GE (1985). Drug Sensitivity Test for
Patients with Acute Leukemia on High Dose AraC
Therapy. Seminars in Oncol 12(2)Supp. 3:31-33.

Perez LM, Mekras JA, Briggle TV, Greer S (1984). Marked
Radiosensitization of Cells in Culture ot X-ray by
5-Chlorodeoxycytidine Coadministered with Tetrahydrouridine and Inhibitors of Pyrimidine Biosynthesis.
Int J Radiat Oncol Biol Phys 10:1453-1458.

Picciano PT, Benedict CV (1986). Mussel Adhesive Protein: A New Cell Attachment Factor. In Vitro Cell
Devel Biol 22(3)Part II:24A.

Plunkett W, Iacoboni SJ, Estey W, Danhauser L, Liliemark JO and Keating MJ (1985). Pharmacologically Directed AraC Therapy for Refractory Leukemia. Seminars in Oncol 12(2)Supp. 3:20-30.

Preisler HD, Rustum YM, Priore RL (1985). Relationship between Leukemic Cell Retention of Cytosine Arabinosylcytosine Triphosphate andthe Duration of Remission in Patients with Acute Nonlymphocytic Leukemia. Europ J Cancer Clin Oncol 21:23-30.

Riccardi R, Chabner B, Glaubiger DL, Wood J, Poplack DG (1982). Influence of Tetrahydrouridine on the Pharmacokinetics of Intrathecally Administered 1-ß-D-Arabinofuranosylcytosine. Cancer Res 42:1736-1739.

Riva C, Rustum YM, Preisler HD (1985). Pharmacokinetics and Cellular Determinants of Response to 1-ß-D-Arabinofuranosylcytosine (AraC). Seminars in Oncol 12(2):1-8.

Riva CM, Rustum YM (1985). 1-ß-D-Arabinofuranosyl-cytosine Metabolism and Incorporation into DNA as Determinants of in vivo Murine Tumor Cell Response. Cancer Res 45:6244-6249.

Rockwell S (1985). Effects of Clumps and Clusters on Survival Measurements with Clonogenic Assays. Cancer Res 45:1601-1607.

Rustum Y, Mayhew E, Szoka F, Campbell J (1981). Inability of Liposome-encapsulated AraC Nucleotides to Overcome AraC Resistance of L1210 Cells. Europ J Cancer 17:809-817.

Rustum YM (1978). Metabolism and Intracellular Retention of Arabinosylcytosine: Predictors of Response of Animal Tumors. Cancer Res 38:543-549.

Rustum YM, Preisler HD (1979). Correlation between Cell Retention of 1-ß-D-Arabinosylcytosine-5'-triphosphate and Response to Therapy. Cancer Res 39:42-49.

Rustum YM, Preisler HD (1979). Correlation between Leukemic Cell Retention of 1-ß-D-arabinosylcytosine-5'-Triphosphate and Response to Therap. Cancer Res 39:42-49.

Rustum YM, Preisler HD (1987). Pharmacokinetic Parameters of 1-ß-D-Arabinofuranosylcytosine (AraC) and their Relationship to Intracellular Metabolism of AraC, Toxicity and Response of Patients with Acute Nonlymphocytic Leukemia (ANLL) Treated with Conventional and High Dose AraC. Seminars in Oncol submitted.

Rustum YM, Slocum HK, Wang G, Bakshi D, Kelly E, Buscaglia D, Wrzosek C, Preisler H (1982). Relationship between Plasma AraC and Intracellular AraCTP Pools under Conditios of Continuous Infusion and High-Dose AraC Treatment. Medical and Pediatric Oncol 1:33-43.

Salmon SF (1980). "Cloning of Human Tumor Stem Cells." New York: Alan R. Liss.

Semple TU, Quinn LA, Woods LK Moore GE (1978). Tumor and Lymphoid Cell Lines from a Patient with Carcinoma of the Colon for a Cytotoxicity Model. Cancer Res 38:1345-1355.

Slocum HK, Greco WR, Parsons J and Rustum YM. An application of image analysis in cancer research. In Absolom DR and Karcich K (eds): "A Practical Guide to Image Analysis," New York Marcel-Dekker, Inc., in preparation.

Slocum HK, Heppner GH, Rustum YM. Cellular heterogeneity of human tumors: Implications for understanding and treating cancer. In Mihich E (ed): "Biological Responses in Cancer," New York: Plenum Press.

Slocum HK, Pavelic ZP, Greco WR, Rustum YM (1984). The Roles of Aggregates in Soft Agar Colony Formation Assays. Proc Am Assoc Cancer Pes 25:377 (Abst. No. 1496).

Smith HS, Lan S, Ceriani P, Hackett AJ (1981). Clonal Proliferation of Cultured Nonmalignant and Malignant Human Breast Epithelia. Cancer Res 41:4637-4643.

Stampfer M, Hallowes RC, Hackett AJ (1980). Growth of Normal Human Mammary Cells in Culture. In Vitro 16(5):415-425.

Thomson SP, Moon TE, Meyskens FL, Jr (1984). Kinetics of Clonogenic Melanoms Cell Proliferation and the Limits on Growth Within a Bilayer Agar System. J Cell Physiol 121:114-124.

Verhoef V, Fridland A. (1986). Alternate Pathways for AraCTP Catabolism in Human Tand B-Lymphoblasts. Proc Am Assoc Cancer Pes 27:299.

Yang J, Guzman R, Richards J, Nandi S (1980). Primary Culture of Mouse Mammary Tumor epithelial Cells Embedded in Collagen Gels. In Vitro 16(6):502-506.

Prediction of Response to Cancer Therapy, pages 139-204
© 1988 Alan R. Liss, Inc.

THE 6-DAY SUBRENAL CAPSULE ASSAY (SRCA): ITS CRITICISM,
BIOLOGY AND REVIEW OF ASSAY/CLINICAL CORRELATIONS.

Arthur E. Bogden, William R. Cobb and Doreen J.
LePage
Biomeasure Incorporated/Bogden Laboratories
11-15 "E" Avenue, Hopkinton, Massachusetts 01748

INTRODUCTION

This chapter will (a) review the basic
biology of the 6-day SRCA which permits use of a
simple tumor size parameter and human tumor
xenografts implanted in conventional murine hosts,
(b) illustrate and discuss the criticism of using
immunologically competent animals, and (c) review
the assay/clinical correlations supporting the
conclusion that the 6-day SRCA is clinically
predictive by accurately measuring a biological
property of the tumor rather than a non-specific
host effect.

The SRCA was designed for testing developmental therapeutic agents against human tumor
xenografts prepared from the solid malignancies
(6). Fundamental to the design were two considerations, (a) that solid tumors are composed of
heterogeneous cell populations in terms of
biosynthetic functions, growth potential and drug
sensitivity, and (b) that the complexity of
epithelial/stromal relationship affects both tumor
growth as well as drug sensitivities. By utilizing a tumor fragment for subrenal capsule
implantation, cell membrane integrity, cell-to-
cell contact, and the spatial relationship of the
cell populations and tissues within the fragment
are maintained permitting the measurement of tumor

response to drug activity as a net response of multiple cell populations, both clonogenic and non-clonogenic. Thus, a degree of heterogeneity in the tissues comprising the xenografts is not only to be expected but is desirable if the fragment to be implanted is a representative fraction of a patients tumor. Selection of the tissue for subcapsular implantation in the SRCA is of prime importance.

SRCA methodology was first applied with transplantation established human tumor xenograft systems utilizing the immunodeficient athymic nude mouse. The assay was of 11-days duration and is utilized by the United States' National Cancer Institute for screening new drugs in lieu of the relatively long term (60-90 days) subcutaneous xenograft assay (33).

The decision to examine the feasibility of substituting the relatively inexpensive normal immunocompetent mouse as xenograft host for drug testing, and abbreviating the assay time frame to six days to avoid artifacts of an immune response, was motivated by the consideration that if transplantable human tumors were to be economically practicable in large scale drug screening programs, even greater economies of time and costs were needed. The cost of the athymic nude mouse and the expense of maintaining a biocontainment housing facility was also prohibitive if the SRCA was to be applied clinically as an individually predictive test.

Feasibility of utilizing the conventional immunocompetent mouse in a 6-day SRCA has been demonstrated at both the preclinical and clinical levels. Sensitivity, reproducibility and predictive quality have been excellent and will be reviewed in the latter part of this chapter.

IS HOST CELL RESPONSE ARTIFACTUAL - A CRITIQUE OF THE CRITICISM

Criticism of the 6-day SRCA is based upon the

microscopic observations of host cell infiltration
of human tumor xenografts six days after implantation under the renal capsule of immunocompetent
mice, suggesting that such infiltration could
contribute to size changes in the xenografts which
could complicate interpretation of chemosensitivity data obtained in the assay.

Edelstein, et al (15) were the first to
report their microscopic observations of the
variable amounts of host cell infiltration in
primary and transplantable human tumor xenografts
on day 6 of the assay period. Unfortunately, in
making what is presented as a "critique of the
method" the authors did not duplicate the drug
doses, regimen and routes of administration
recommended by Bogden; calculated test results on
the basis of percent control surface area,
definitely not recommended by Bogden; and rather
than reporting actual change in tumor size, they
reported a relative tumor size, complicating valid
compar- isons with data in publications utilizing
SRCA methodology.

Table 1 compares the drug doses and treatment
regimens recommended by Bogden with the modifications by Edelstein. Day 1 and 5 treatment
regimen in the 6-day SRCA is the least effective
as compared to a QD1-5, a Day 1 and 3 or a Day 1,
2 and 3 (12). Such a relatively ineffective
regimen could very well explain Edelstein's
inability to induce a response to Cisplatin and
Adriamycin in ovarian cancers.

Edelstein, et al (15) present several tables
illustrating tumor response to drugs as percent
control surface area and the corresponding
estimated microscopic contribution of tumor cells
and host resistance cells to the tumor mass. They
conclude that host cell infiltration causes the
discrepancy between macroscopic and microscopic
evaluation. In Table 2 we have taken Edelstein's
data from page 998 of his publication (15) and
ranked the 12 cytoxan treated ovarian tumors
according to size, i.e., % control surface area,

TABLE 1

DIFFERENCES IN DRUG DOSES AND TREATMENT REGIMENS

Drugs Tested	Dose/Regimen/Route/(Total Dose) Bogden	Edelstein
Cytoxan	50mg/kg, QD1 5, s.c. (250)	200mg/kg, D1 and 5, s.c. (400)
Cisplatin	3mg/kg, QD1-5, s.c. (15)	8mg/kg, D1 and 5, i.v. (16)
Adriamycin	5mg/kg, QD1-5, i.v. (25)	10mg/kg, D1 and 5, i.v. (20)
5-Fluorouracil	50mg/kg, QD1-5, s.c. (250)	175mg/kg, D1 and 5, i.v. (350)

TABLE 2

HISTOLOGICAL ANALYSIS OF TUMOR AND/OR HOST TISSUES IN THE SUBRENAL
CAPSULE TECHNIQUE IN UNTREATED CONTROL AND CYTOXAN TREATED MICE AFTER 6-DAYS

Tumor	Test Results % Control Surface Area[+]	Relative Contribution of: 1 Control Tumor Cells	2 Control Host Cells	3 Cytoxan Treated Tumor Cells
Ovarian L/2	85	+	+++	++++
Ovarian G/1	85	++	++	++
Ovarian U/1	79	+	±	±
Ovarian V/1	70	++	++	+
Ovarian F/1	69	++	+	+
Ovarian P/2	64	++	+	±
Ovarian A/3	61	++	+	+++
Ovarian T/1	58	++	++	+
Ovarian E/3	57	++	++	++++
Ovarian 24/1	38	++	++	+
Ovarian S/3	28	++	+	++
Ovarian 25/1	20	+++	+++	++

[+] Data extracted from Table 2, page 998, reference article by Edelstein (15), rearranged by tumor size (% control surface area) from top to bottom.

Note: Figure after the tumor code represents the passage of the tumor.

largest (85%) at the top to smallest (20%) at the
bottom. We have included the relative contribution of tumor cells (column 1) and host cells
(column 2) to control xenografts, as well as the
relative contribution of tumor cells to cytoxan
treated xenografts (column 3). It is of interest
to point out that the contribution of tumor cells
in control xenografts on day 6 is relatively the
same whether the donor tumor was of primary origin
or had been passaged. There appears to be no
correlation between the estimated relative
contribution of tumor cells in cytoxan treated
tumor xenografts (column 3) and tumor size.
However, there is also no correlation between host
response as indicated by control host cells
(column 2) and the relative contribution of tumor
cells to control xenografts (column 1). Although
the relative contribution of tumor cells in control xenografts is fairly consistent from tumor to
tumor (column 1) host cell response is variable.
Significantly there is no correlation between host
response as indicated by the relative contribution
of control host cells (column 2) and response of
the ovarian tumors to cytoxan.

Since cytoxan was presumably active therapeutically as well as immunosuppressive in the
xenografted animals, we examined the histological
responses to cisplatin as presented by Edelstein
in the same publication (15).

In Table 3 we have also ranked the cisplatin
treated tumors and their corresponding data
according to tumor size i.e., from the largest
(top) to the smallest (bottom). In this table,
however, we have added the relative contributions
of host cells to cisplatin treated xenografts
(column 4), since the drug was presumably inactive
and not immunosuppressive. Presented in this
fashion there is obviously no correlation between
the relative contribution of cisplatin treated
tumor cells (column 3) and degree of host cell
infiltration of the treated tumors (column 4) and
that of tumor size on day 6. The degree of host
cell infiltration (column 2) also does not appear

TABLE 3

HISTOLOGICAL ANALYSIS OF TUMOR AND/OR HOST TISSUES IN THE SUBRENAL CAPSULE TECHNIQUE IN UNTREATED CONTROL AND CISPLATIN TREATED MICE AFTER 6-DAYS

Tumor	Test Results % Control Surface Area[+]	Relative Contribution of:		Cisplatin Treated	
		Control Tumor Cells	Control Host Cells	Tumor Cells[3]	Host Cells[4]
Ovarian S/3	146	++	+	+	++
Ovarian U/1	133	++	-	+	±
Ovarian A/3	126	++	+	+	++
Ovarian 24/1	119	++	++	+++	+
Ovarian G/1	115	++	++	+	++
Ovarian F/1	108	++	+	+	++
Ovarian E/3	101	++	++	++	+++
Ovarian T/1	99	++	++	++	++
Ovarian P/2	98	++	+	±	++
Ovarian 25/1	97	+++	+++	+	++
Ovarian L/2	92	+	+++	+	++
Ovarian V/1	75	++	++	+	+++

[+]Data extracted from Table 2, page 998, reference article by Edelstein (15), rearranged by tumor size (% control surface area) from top to bottom.

to affect the relative contribution of tumor cells in untreated controls on day 6.

In their study the authors have examined tumor xenografts at only one time point in the assay and assumed that the host cellular response observed was artifactual to a tumor size parameter. On the basis of xenograft sizes obtained on only two tumors implanted in athymic nude and normal mice (Table 4) they further conclude that host cell infiltration increases the size of the 6-day xenograft. When reporting responsiveness of two ovarian tumors to cytostatics in normal and nude mice, Edelstein compared first and second passages of the tumor in normal mice to tumors in the sixth and eighth passages in the nude, a comparison of questionable validity.

In a second publication (16) Edelstein, et al, examined several immunosuppressive forms of pretreatment in normal mice in an effort to reduce host cell response in the 6-day SRCA. Drug doses, routes of administration and treatment regimen for normal mice were the same as in the previous study. Because of increased sensitivity to drug toxicity, nude mice were treated only on day 1. This difference in the day of treatment is important to note because the authors observed that there was a significant difference between control and treated tumors on day 6 that was found in the nude mouse and which was not found in the normal mouse. They attribute the apparent loss of sensitivity in the normal mouse to the extra "growth" representing ingrowth of host response cells. However, in a comparison of treatment schedules in the 6-day SRCA Cobb, et al (12), showed that the antitumor effect of a single injection of drug was greatest when administered on day 1 post tumor implantation. When the same total dose was divided into two injections, the most effective treatments were those which were administered on days 1 and 2, or on days 1 and 3. Edelstein's assumption is not substantiated and his interpretation of the relative sensitivity as an artifact of host cell infiltration is invalid.

TABLE 4

MEAN GROWTH (SURFACE AREA) OF TUMOR UNDER THE

RENAL CAPSULE AFTER 6 DAYS*

Ovarian Tumor	Immunocompetent 'normal'		Immunodeficient 'nude'
X Ov. P	1.95+0.107	p<0.01	1.38+0.1007
X Ov. S	2.11+0.135	n.s.	1.32+0.76

*Data from Table 5, page 1008, reference article by Edelstein (15).

TABLE 5

COMPARISON OF THE INCREASE IN SIZE OF HUMAN OVARIAN TUMOR

XENOGRAFTS AND THE DEGREE OF HOST CELL INFILTRATION[1]

Tumor Code	Relative Tumor Growth $(mm)^2$	Degree of Infiltration	Tumor Cells %
37	+0.10	+	60
30	+0.10	+ +	50
38	+0.11	+ +	45
33	+0.19	+ + +	0
34	+0.20	+	60
29	+0.24	+ + +	0
31	+0.38	+ +	60
32	+0.39	+ +	0
39	+0.46	- - -	85
36	+0.52	+	55
35	+0.57	+ +	50

[1]Data excerpted from reference article by Edelstein (16).

[2]Change in tumor size in the 6-day SRCA. Fresh surgical explants.

In the same study (16), the authors found that whole body irradiation, though preferred for immunosuppression, did not completely prevent cellular infiltration of primary tumors. Relative tumor growth was determined on eleven human ovarian tumors on day 6 and the percentage of tumor cells as well as host cell infiltration was estimated microscopically. The authors found no correlation between growth of the xenografts and percentage tumor cells, again suggesting an artificatual role for host cell infiltration.

In Table 5, we have taken this same ovarian data and arranged relative tumor growth in order of the smallest tumor at the top to the largest at the bottom. There obviously is no correlation between tumor size and percent of tumor cells. However, there is also no correlation between the degree of host cell infiltration and percent of tumor cells or tumor size. A relationship between the degree of host cell infiltration and change in tumor size over the 6-day assay period has not been established other than to demonstrate evidence of host cell infiltration on day 6.

We would suggest that some variability and lack of correlation of microscopic and macroscopic observations is due to the innate difficulties in preparing histological sections of 1.0mm cubed fragments of tumor that would provide a truly representative microscopic picture when only a single section is cut and examined. We have found that, where on the tumor fragment a cut is made, and how many cuts are made, markedly influence the results of microscopic analysis, see Figure 1.

Edelstein expresses surprise that even in the nude mouse, no tumor is composed only of tumor cells, and confesses that "part of the hetero-geneity seen in the histological sections on day 6 can be found prior to implantation in the 1mm^3 tumor pieces" (16). He concludes, however, that this intrinsic heterogeneity of most but not all tumors is undesirable if bulk growth and bulk

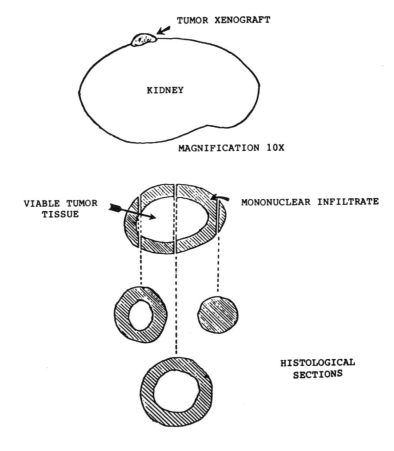

Figure 1. The variability in tumor/host cell ratios that can be obtained when preparing random histological sections of subcapsularly implanted 1.0mm cubed fragments of tumor tissue.

reduction are the parameters of tumor response. The practicability of the SRCA is use of the tumor fragment. Tumor heterogeneity is an accepted fact. Forty to 60 tumor fragments are selected at random as a sampling of the patient's tumor for SRCA. If the fragments are to predict for the response of the patient's tumor they must be representative of the patient's tumor, be it homogeneous or heterogeneous. That selection of the tissue for subcapsular implantation in the SRCA is of prime importance cannot be overemphasized. Preselection control is feasible and will be discussed later in this chapter.

Bennett, et al (5) examined fresh surgical explants of human carcinomas as first transplant generation xenografts after 6 days under the renal capsule of normal immunocompetent mice, immunodeficient athymic nude mice and immunosuppressed conventional mice. They reported significant host cell infiltration of human tumor xenografts implanted in normal mice suggesting that this microscopically evidenced infiltrate could contribute to artifactual size changes in the SRCA. However, in contrast to Edelstein's conclusions that host cell response artifactually increased the size of xenografts in normal mice, Bennett concluded that tumors grew better in the immunocompromised animal, and that host response was inhibitory to tumor growth by day 6 of the assay period.

The major criticism of this study lies in the fact that most tumor size data was obtained from only one or two animals at a time point and is presented in tabular form as means +/- range of two values. As evidence in support of their conclusions, the authors compared the size changes (ΔTS) occurring with fresh surgical explants after 6 days under the renal capsule of normal and athymic nude mice. They observed that there was no correlation between the amount of tumor detectable microscopically and change in xenograft size in athymic nudes. In all cases, the amount of tumor in the xenograft was less in immunocompetent mice than it was in nude mice with significant infiltration around the tumor in the immunologically competent animal. They do acknowledge, however, that there was also some infiltration by mononuclear cells in human colon xenografts implanted in the athymic nudes. This data is presented in Table 1 of their publication (5).

Also evident, but not discussed by Bennett, is the lack of correlation between the amount of tumor detectable microscopically and change of xenograft size in the normal immunocompetent animal. In Table 6 we have compared Bennett's data on xenograft changes in normal and athymic nude mice over the 6 day assay period. In consideration that each of the ΔTS values represents the mean of only two xenografts, and the same tumor was implanted in both normal and corresponding nude pairs, we compared overall tumor growth in athymic and normal mice by averaging the ΔTS values of the seven colon tumors. The averaged ΔTS value for each group of animals is shown at the bottom of Table 6. The average 0.12mm growth for each group strongly suggests that the growth potential of the colon tumor xenografts was comparable whether implanted in normal or athymic nude hosts. Xenograft size in the normal and athymic nude mouse on day 6 represents the growth potential of the tissue implanted on day 0. However, the differences, as noted between individual animals implanted with tissue from the same donor, may be due to the inherent variability in implantation technique and measurements when only 2 animals are used per time point. This suggestion is reinforced by the data for all ten tumors which shows that the ΔTS of 5 tumors out of ten was greater in normal mice than in the corresponding athymic nudes, and by the same token, the ΔTS of 5 tumors out of ten was greater in athymic nude mice than in the corresponding normal mice.

The final bit of Bennett's data that does not support his conclusion that xenograft growth is

TABLE 6

HUMAN TUMOR XENOGRAFT CHANGES IN 6-DAY XENOGRAFTS IMPLANTED

UNDER THE KIDNEY CAPSULE OF NORMAL AND NUDE MICE

The data shown are the mean of only two mice $\pm$ the range from two

mice.

Patient	Tumor	Normal ΔTS (mm)	Nude ΔTS (mm)
1	Colon Adenocarcinoma	+0.1$\pm$0.2	+0.45$\pm$0.05
2	Colon Adenocarcinoma	-0.02$\pm$0.07	-0.1$\pm$0.1
3	Colon Adenocarcinoma	+0.07$\pm$0.08	-0.02$\pm$0.02
4	Colon Adenocarcinoma	+0.05$\pm$0.2	+0.2$\pm$0.2
5	Colon Adenocarcinoma	+0.37$\pm$0.07	+0.13$\pm$0.07
6	Colon Adenocarcinoma	+0.42$\pm$0.02	+0.22$\pm$0.16
7	Colon Adenocarcinoma	-0.1$\pm$0.05	0.0$\pm$0.05
8	Esophageal Squam. Cell	+0.1	+0.17$\pm$0.08
9	Lung Adenocarcinoma	+0.4$\pm$0.1	-0.05$\pm$0.1
10	Head & Neck Squam. Cell	0$\pm$0.1	+0.22$\pm$0.02

Average growth of colon tumors	=	0.89/7	0.88/7
		0.127 mm	0.125 mm

ALL TUMORS:

ΔTS in normal < nude = 5

ΔTS in normal > nude = 5

better in the immunocompromised than in the immunocompetent animal for the first 6 days, is a comparison of the persistence and growth of human colon cancer xenografts under the renal capsule of immunocompetent and immunodeficient mice over a 15 day period. Immunodeficient mice consisted of athymic nude mice; thymectomized, irradiated, bone-marrow-reconstituted mice (TIB), and mice treated with cyclosporin.

We are certainly in agreement with Bennett, et al (5), that host rejection in the normal mouse after day 6 produces a size artifact (tumors begin to regress) and that xenografts in immunocompromised animals continue to increase in size. Our concern, however, is the relative tumor size measurements on day 6.

In Table 7 we have compared the ΔTS values of the human colon tumor xenografts obtained in normal mice and in the various immunocompromised mice over a nine day period. This is Bennett's data taken from Table 2 of his publication (5). The validity of the data is questionable since each data point represents the mean +/- range obtained from measurements made on only two animals. By day 3 post implantation, tumor growth was measurable in normal mice (too early for rejection) and immunocompromised TIB mice; one tumor grew and one tumor showed regression in the athymic nudes; and no tumors grew in cyclosporin immunosuppressed mice. On day 6, tumor growth, as indicated by a + ΔTS, was evident in normal mice and in athymic mice. There was no growth in immunocompromised TIB mice, and actual tumor regression in mice treated with cyclosporin. The erratic data obtained with sequential measurements would indicate (a) a large range in measuring error and (b) heterogeneity in the quality of tumor xenografts implanted in the various groups. Nonetheless, the data certainly indicate that, within the 6 day time-frame, tumor xenografts do not necessarily grow better in the immunocompromised animal.

In a more recent study by Abrams, et al (4), the 6-day SRCA was performed in normal mice using fresh surgical explants of non small cell lung and ovarian cancers. Multiagent chemotherapy combinations were evaluated for activity against these two tumor types. Macroscopic results (tumor size) measured via an ocular microscope showed high activity for some combinations as well as for single agents. The assay was able to discriminate drug sensitivity of different tumors. However, when subjected to microscopic examination, they reported that the SRC implants in the untreated control animals did not show viable tumor growth on day 6 and there was an inflammatory and fibrotic reaction in the majority of grafts. Following the lead of Edelstein, et al, they drew the conclusion that because of the host response observed on day 6 in untreated control animals, the drug sensitivity patterns obtained by tumor size measurements in treated animals must be artifactual. No attempt was made to compare macroscopic SRCA results with clinical results.

Unfortunately, Abrams, et al, also commit the error of Edelstein and do not administer the recommended drug dose levels as single agents, nor follow the treatment regimen recommended by Bogden (QD1-5) or that used successfully by Aamdal (1), i.e., treatment on days 1 and 2. Table 8 compares the treatment protocol and dose levels recommended by Bogden with that used by Abrams. Note that Bogden administers a 3mg/kg dose, s.c., QD1-5 of cisplatin, and Aamdal administered a dose of 6mg/kg, i.v. on days 1 and 2 (1), with acceptable toxicity. Abrams reports that 3mg/kg, i.v. on days 1 and 2 resulted in unacceptable toxicity because of the trauma of surgery and, therefore changed treatment to days 2 and 3. In view of this modification by Abrams it is not surprising that these investigators, similar to Edelstein, had low response rates to cisplatin.

In Table 9 we have taken the control data from Table 5, 6 and 7 of Abrams, et al, publication (4), and compared the change in tumor size

TABLE 7

PERSISTENCE AND GROWTH OF HUMAN COLON CANCER XENOGRAFTS UNDER THE

RENAL CAPSULE OF NORMAL; NUDE; THYMECTOMIZED, IRRADIATED, BONE-

MARROW-RECONSTITUTED MICE (TIB); AND MICE TREATED WITH CYCOSPORIN

Data is mean + range of two animals

Days After Implantation	Normal ΔTS (mm)	Nude ΔTS (mm)	TIB ΔTS (mm)	Cyclosporin ΔTS (mm)
3	+0.1+0.7	0+0.15	+0.2+0.07	0
6	+0.1+0.2	+0.4+0.05	0	-0.1+0.05
9	-0.2+0.1	+0.7+0.25	+0.4	+0.3+0.2
	Moderate Growth Day 6	Extraordinary Growth Day 6	No Growth Day 6	Regression Day 6

TABLE 8

COMPARISON OF TREATMENT FOR SINGLE AGENTS RECOMMENDED

BY BOGDEN AND THAT USED BY ABRAMS

Chemotherapeutic Agent	Dose, Route and Treatment Regimen Bogden	Abrams
Cisplatin	3mg/kg, s.c., QD1-5 Total Dose: 15mg/kg	3mg/kg, i.v., days 2 and 3 Total Dose: 6mg/kg
VP-16	32mg/kg, s.c., QD1-5 Total Dose: 160mg/kg	30mg/kg, i.v., days 2 and 3 Total Dose: 60mg/kg
L-PAM	6mg/kg, s.c., QD1-5 Total Dose: 30mg/kg	4mg/kg, i.v., days 2 and 3 Total Dose: 8mg/kg

Reference to article by J. Abrams, et al, Eur. J. Cancer Clinical Oncol. 22 (11): 1387-1394, 1986.

TABLE 9

DAY 6 COMPARISON OF CHANGE IN TUMOR SIZE AND THE DEGREE OF INFLAMMATION BY

HOST CELLS AND FIBROSIS IN UNTREATED CONTROL GRAFTS[1]

Exp.	Change In Tumor Size[2]	Degree of Inflammation[3]	Degree of Fibrosis[3]
Lung SRC Grafts			
8	-0.4	+ +	-
30	-0.2	+ + +	+
11	-0.2	+ +	+ +
26	+1.1	+ +	+ +
27	+1.8	+ + +	-
10	+2.0	+ + + +	-
1	+2.0	+ +	-
28	+2.3	+ +	+
29	+2.8	+ + +	+
12	+3.4	+ + +	-
Ovarian SRC Grafts			
13	0.0	+ + +	+
20	0.0	+ +	+
14	+0.5	+ +	+ +
22	+0.8	+	+ +
6	+1.2	+ +	+ +
9	+1.6	+ + +	-
5	+2.0	+ +	-
7	+2.8	+ + + +	-

[1]Data taken from Tables 6 and 7 in reference article by J. Abrams, _et al._ (4)

[2]Change in tumor size (ΔTS) in ocular micrometer units, i.e., 1mm = 10omu

[3]Microscopic code: + = 0-25% total area, ++ = 25-50% total area;
+++ = 50-75% total area; ++++ = 75-100% total area.

with the degree of inflammation by host cells and
fibrosis in untreated control grafts of lung and
ovarian tumors on day 6. Tumors are ranked
according to size. Similar to Edelstein's data,
there is no correlation between xenograft size and
the degree of host response. Nevertheless, tumors
show variation in size that permits their ranking
according to size which we would suggest reflects
individual tumor growth potential. The lack of
correlation between xenograft size and degree of
infiltration does not support the assumption that
host cellular response creates a size artifact.

Table 10 compares the control growth with the
ratio of microscopically detectable tumor in day 0
paired specimens of controls and treated mice.
This data was extracted from several tables in the
Abrams article in an attempt to determine whether
the amount or number of tumor cells, microscopically discernable in control grafts prior to
implantation, was representative of the quality of
tissue implanted in treated animals. Tumors are
ranked by Δ Tumor Size, i.e., largest at the top
to smallest at the bottom. The denominator
indicates the total number of paired tumor
specimens (fragments) examined and the numerator
the number of examined fragments containing tumor
cells. Although the number of tumors examined (5
lung, 2 ovarian) is small, when none of the
control specimens (0 out of 23) showed microscopic
evidence of tumor on day 0 prior to implantation
(SRC No.'s 20 an 30), there was either no change
in xenograft size or there was evidence of
regression. Although, the number of tumor cell
containing specimens, from any particular tumor
observed on day 0, did not correlate with mean
change in tumor size on day 6, there was an
increase in xenograft size as long as there was
some evidence of tumor cells present prior to
implantation.

That control xenograft specimens examined for
microscopic evidence of tumor cells will predict
for the quality of paired xenografts implanted in
treated animals is illustrated on the bottom of

TABLE 10

COMPARISON OF CONTROL GROWTH WITH RATIO OF MICROSCOPICALLY DETECTABLE

TUMOR IN DAY O PAIRED SPECIMENS OF CONTROL AND TREATED MICE

SRC No.	ΔTS (omu)	Controls Tumored/Specimens		Treated Tumored/Specimens	
29	+2.8	1/12	8%	0/15	0%
28	+2.3	3/4	75%	5/12	42%
27	+1.8	7/10	70%	10/15	67%
26	+1.1	3/11	27%	7/12	58%
22*	+0.8	12/12	100%	15/15	100%
20*	0.0	0/12	0%	7/15	47%
30	-0.2	0/11	0%	0/15	0%

Data recompiled from Table 8 in reference article by J. Abrams, et al. (4)

*Ovarian tumors, all others lung tumors

TOTAL PAIRED SPECIMENS OF LUNG TUMOR XENOGRAFTS HAVING

HISTOLOGICALLY PROVEN TUMOR ON DAY O

Controls	Treated
14/48 29%	22/69 32%

Table 10. When 29% (14/48) of paired lung tumor xenografts had histologically proven tumor on day 0, then 32% (22/69) of the corresponding paired specimens selected for implantation into treated animals also had histologically proven tumor.

Abrams points out the variability in tumor content of fresh surgical specimens as a possible negative factor. However, human tumors are heterogenious masses of tissue and specimens for predicitve assays should reflect the heterogeneity of the patient's tumor. That the implantation of "good" tumor tissue can be assured by more fastidious selection and monitoring of speciments for implantations, has been indicated by Abram's data. We would recommend the tissue quality control procedure advocated by Levi, et al (21). On day 0, 10 fragments of tumor are randomly selected from among those to be implanted (5 at the beginning and 5 at the end of the procedure). These are fixed in Bouin's solution, cryostat sectioned, or fluorescense stained and processed for histologic analysis. The assay is considered valid if 7 of the 10 fragments contain tumor cells.

WHY THE DETAILED ANALYSIS OF NEGATIVE REPORTS

The four publications critiqued in this report (15, 16, 5, 4) originate from three investigative groups. They were selected for detailed analysis because their publications represent the bulk and are typical of the negative criticisms of the 6-day SRCA. Also, we felt that it was important to show that the negative conclusions that have been drawn were based, primarily, on assumption, and that none of the critical investigative groups compared macroscopic SRCA results with clinical responses, even retrospectively. The excellent SRCA/clinical correlations obtained in several medical centers in the United States and Europe have been ignored. One group (4) critiqued in this report made no mention of an earlier publication (14) from their institution in which the sensitivity of 24 malignant melanomas to six chemotherapeutic agents was examined in the 6-day SRCA using the tumor size parameter. The evaluable assay rate was reported as 95% with a fair correlation between "microscopic" and "macroscopic" parameters. Most importantly, good correlations were obtained between the percentage of responses in the 6-day SRCA and that of clinical responses for the same drugs (Table 11).

Implantation of human tissue, albeit malignant and under the renal capsule, is somewhat of an unorthodox procedure immunologically. Studies, such as those critiqued in this report, have a bias in that they are designed to demonstrate why the assay should not be feasible rather than the mechanism of its feasibility. None of the laboratories duplicated exactly the recommended procedure nor attempted to correlate assay results with clinical responses. Untreated control xenografts have been examined, primarily, on day 6 at the end of the assay period, and the expected host cellular responses described. On the basis of these microscopic observations in the control xenografts, the assumption has been made that the "tumor size" parameter may be an artifact and therefore, the immunocompetent animal cannot be validly used in the 6-day SRCA. None of the critiqued laboratories carried out actual quantitative measurements of size and cell number. Such objective measurements have been made by only one group, Aamdal, Fodstad and Phil (2), who concluded "the mouse cell infiltration is clearly of little consequence for the measurement of growth."

NECROSIS AND FUNCTION OF CONTROL XENOGRAFTS

Early in the development of the 6-day SRCA varying degrees of cellular response were evident in and around untreated tumor xenografts beginning about day 4 of the assay period. It was evident, moreover, that the change in size of the tumor xenograft during the 6-day assay period was the result of many factors intrinsic to both the host and the implanted tissue.

TABLE 11

COMPARISON OF RESPONSE RATES IN THE SUBRENAL CAPSULE ASSAY

TO SINGLE AGENT CHEMOTHERAPY IN PUBLISHED CLINICAL TRAILS:

MALIGNANT MELONOMA

Drugs Tested	Clinical Experience[1]	SRC Assay[2]
L-PAM	16	16
DTIC	23	28
Cisplatin	14	14
TGU[3]	Not Known	31
VDS[4]	17	16
BCNU	17	27

[1]Bellet et al. In: W.H. Clark, L.I. Goldman and M.J.
Mastrangelo (eds.), Human Malignant Melanoma, pp. 325-341,
Grune & Stratton, New York (1979).

[2]Dumont, P. et al. Int. J. Cancer 33: 447-451 (1984).
Institute Jules Bordet and Netherlands Cancer Institute.

[3]TGU = triglycidyl urazol

[4]Vindesine sulphate

When non-necrotic, non-infected, fresh viable tumor tissue is implanted subcapsularly, one observes an increase in xenograft size that is directly related to the mitotic activity observed in the original tumor specimen (7). Necrosis, whether inherent in the tumor or induced intentionally by a chemical agent, is quickly resorbed from the subcapsular site. Therefore, tumor size on day 6 is the result of cell division and resorption of non-viable cells. Histology of the untreated xenograft on day 6, then, reflects (a) the quality of tissue implanted and (b) the resultant interactions of tumor cells and host tissues. Importantly, host response is _proportional_ to the amount of viable malignant tissue implanted and the persistence of such tissue to the end of the assay period, the former influencing the strength and the latter influencing persistence of the antigenic stimulus. The point being made is that assuming healthy malignant tissue has been implanted, the histologic picture of untreated xenografts on day 6 can only reflect the accumulative effect of tumor-host interaction. It is emphasized that tumor cell synthesis of extracellular matrix components and the increased production of matrix components by host cells in response to the presence of the xenograft are phenomena associated with _viable_ tumor cells.

Since chemotherapy is initiated early in the assay period, i.e., day 1, drug sensitive tumor cells are necrotized early. As a result, the number of tumor cells surviving to day 6 is proportional to the sensitivity of the tumor to the test drug, and the reduction in the mass and viability of tumor tissue at the implant site is reflected by a proportional reduction of the tumor/host mediated responses at that site. One cannot assume that certain histological features evident in control xenografts on day 6 of the assay period are artifactual to a tumor size parameter or do not represent a quantitative response of the xenograft to chemotherapy.

It must be stressed, that the SRCA was designed to mimic the clinical situation in that the inital in situ tumor xenograft measurement provides each tumor with its own base line for evaluating drug effects. The final size of the control does not provide a numerical value for evaluating drug effects in the treated animal. As in the clinic, for a tumor to be considered responsive to drug treatment, it must show a measurable regression in size i.e., a-ΔTS. Drug activity in the assay is measured as an oncolytic effect. Although an increase in the size of control xenografts on day 6 reflects the growth potential of the donor tumor, control size is used only to indicate the quality of tissue that was implanted. Untreated xenografts laced with necrosis will show a wide variability in final size as well as regressions. A mean-ΔTS in the control indicates excessive necrosis in the tumor sample and thus flags the unevaluable assay (7).

SRCA DESIGN AND BIOLOGY IN SUPPORT OF THE 6-DAY SRCA

The following discussion concerns the design and biology of the SRCA relevant to the feasibility of a 6-day time frame and the use of the conventional normal, immunocompetent mouse as host for human tumor xenografts.

The basic questions (a) does malignant human tissue "grow" when implanted under the renal capsule of normal, immunocompetent mice, and (b) is the host cellular infiltration evident on day 6 in untreated control animals, artifactual to a simple tumor size parameter for evaluating drug effect in treated animals, have been objectively examined in several laboratories.

The most objective and quantitative studies on the growth of human tumor xenografts implanted under the renal capsule of conventional mice and host immune response, have been carred out by Aamdal, et al (2, 3) at the Norsk Hydro's Institute for Cancer Research in Oslo. The growth of 29 different human tumor lines which included malignant melanomas, colon carcinomas, soft tissue sarcomas, lung cancers and mammary carcinomas implanted under the renal capsule of immunocompetent mice, was investigated.

All tumors showed distinct growth within 2-4 days demonstrating little or no lag time which was supported by the observation that on day 2 there was already a high mitotic rate. Xenografts generally stopped growing after day 6. If the animals were immunosuppressed by pretreatment with cyclophosphamide, tumor growth did not stop on day 6 but continued at the same rate for 2 more days. Importantly, it appears that pretreatment (immunosuppression) did not increase the growth rate of the grafts during the first 6 days, indicating that the host immune response did not measurably inhibit the growth rate during the assay period. Reproducibility of the growth measured was determined by repeated measurements carried out over a period of several years on 17 human tumor xenografts of different tumor types. It was found that the growth rates of subcapsularly implanted tumors remained constant with time and that for all tumor types tested the xenografts showed different and individual growth rates for up to 6 days. When the growth rates of subcapsular grafts in the normal murine host were compared with those observed when the same tumors were growing subcutaneously in athymic nude mice, the relative growth rates were pratically the same in the two systems. The results indicate that the growth conditions under the renal capsule of normal mice permits the expression of inherent growth potentials. That tumor cells retained their malignant character for 6 days under the renal capsule of immunocompetent mice was demonstrated by the observation that when grafts were removed from the kidneys after 6-days, single cell suspensions were able to form colonies in soft agar and to form subcutaneous tumors in athymic nude mice.

The aspect of host cell infiltration was also

thoroughly investigated by this group. Not only did human tumor xenografts grow well under the renal capsule of immunocompetent mice, but they retained morphological and functional character- istics of the parent tumors, as judged by light and electron microscopy and immunohistochemical examinations. Numerous mitoses were detected. Granulation tissue and necrosis were not predominant features. Grafts became infiltrated from the periphery by mouse inflammatory cells after day 4 (3).

The extent of infiltration of the grafts by host cells was measured by flow cytometry on single cell suspensions as well as by quantitative analysis of serial histological sections (2). The results of flow cytometric measurements carried out on a number of different tumors indicated that as many as 28-60% of the cells were actually mouse cells. Interestingly, when athymic nude mice were used as host animals, as many as 28% of the cells in the subcapsular graft on day 6 consisted of mouse cells.

Since the inflammatory mouse cells are considerably smaller than the human tumor cells the extent of infiltration of the graft by mouse cells and their potential contribution to zenograft size, was also assessed histologically. Serial sections (3μ thick) were cut at intervals of 100 to 300μ and stained with H&E. The area of the entire graft and the areas occupied by mouse and human tumor tissue were identified, delineated and estimated by use of a semi-automatic quantitative image analyzer. The results for 9 tumors showed that in most cases the mouse cells occupied about 15-35% of the total graft volume on day 6. Thus, the presence of, e.g., 25 volume percent of mouse cells would cause a difference in the measured diameters of the grafts of only about 7-10%, which is within measuring error of the procedure. Aamdal, et al concluded that the results suggest that the 6-day SRCA in immunocompetent mice is adequate for practical purposes (2).

The subcapsular site provides a naturally rich, vascular bed which permits unrestricted delivery of nutrients as well as test drugs to the implanted tissue. Mitotic and biosynthetic activity of newly implanted tumor xenografts continue unabated with no anoxic lag time as with subcutaneously implanted tumors awaiting vascularization. Furthermore, initial implantation of a $1.0mm^3$ tumor fragment provides no barriers to the diffusion of gasses, nutrients and test drugs throughout the tumor.

Sands, et al (28) compared blood perfusion of murine and human tumor xenografts implanted s.c. and under the renal capsule of normal and athymic nude mice. Tumor blood flow was measured indirectly by fractional distribution of 86 Rubidium Chloride. They found that subcapsular implanted tumors showed between 5-7 times greater blood flow than subcutaneous tumors.

Price, in collaborative studies at the University of Massachusetts Medical Center (unpublished data), examined for the presence and viability of tumor cells in gynecologic tumors implanted subcapsularly in normal mice over a 12 day period using ^{3}H-thymidine uptake in a standard autoradiographic technique. In corroboration of Aamdal's observations with transplantable human tumors, Price found that thymidine uptake by tumor xenografts of both transplantable and fresh surgical explants increased following implantation, peaking on day 4 or 5. Though diminished, thymidine uptake by tumor cells was still evident at the end of the 6-day assay period. Host cell response, on the other hand, peaked about days 10 or 12.

The peaking of proliferative activity observed in human tumor xenografts on day 4 or 5 correlates with the histologic observations of Levi, et al (21). Fragments of fresh explants of human tumors were found to retain their proliferative and metabolic capacity for at least

4 days after implantation under the renal capsule of immunocompetent mice. This was indicated by the mitosis in xenografts, that of keratinizing cells in xenografts from epidermoid carcinoma, and that of melanin producing cells in xenografted melanomas. In some tumor specimens capillaries filled with mouse erythrocytes were observed in xenografts sampled on day 4. During this time frame, only minimal, if any, lymphocytic infiltration was observed at the limit between the tumor and the renal tubules. These investigators found the overall quality of tumor xenografts on day 4 adequately preserved to establish histological scoring of treated and control xenografts as the parameters for evaluating drug effects in a 4-day assay. The integrity of the tumor cells is further supported by the high uptake of monoclonal antibodies by freshly explanted human tumors 3 and 4 days after implantation under the renal capsule in immunocompetent mice (8).

Levi (21) noted that the extent of lymphyocytic infiltration of the xenograft though minimal on day 4, invaded the entire xenograft by day 6. Nevertheless, of 44 untreated xenografts studied, the mean change in tumor size (ΔTS) of xenografts from any tumor specimen did not differ between days 4 and 6 (p>0.10). This observation is extremely important because days 5 and 6 are obviously the time frame in the 6-day SRCA of greatest host cell infiltration.

The fact that the extensive host cell infiltration of human tumor xenografts, occurring on days 5 and 6, resulted in no significant increases in xenograft size correlates with the quantitative observations of Aamdal (2, 3), and explains the lack of correlation between the degree of host cell infiltration and tumor size on day 6 in the data reported by Edelstein (16), Bennett (5) and Abrams (4).

Relative to the importance for careful selection of the tissue to be implanted, Levi, et al (21) found a statistically significant (p<0.001) correlation between the rate of fragments containing cancer cells in the quality control test and the rate of xenografts containing cancer cells on day 4. Thus, good viable tissue can be preselected for implantation. When non-necrotic, non-infected, fresh viable tumor tissue is implanted subcapsularly one observes an increase in untreated xenografts size that is directly related to the mitotic activity (growth potential) of the original tumor specimen (7). The size of treated xenografts, on the other hand, is the resultant of mitotic activity and drug induced cell death, drug resistance favoring continued growth and drug sensitivity favoring oncolysis.

Evidence supporting the viability of human tumor xenografts (fresh surgical explants) during the critical time frame of the 6-day SRCA, has also been reported by several other investigators. Realizing the problem of adequate histologic sampling of $1.0mm^3$ size grafts, Reale (26) compared the histologic pattern of fresh surgical explants of human tumors implanted subcapsularly in normal and athymic nude mice over a period of 6 to 10 days by sectioning kidneys up to 30 levels. After a double blind study of over 1500 slides, he concluded that (a) tumor histologic architecture is preserved in explants out to day 6; (b) host infiltrates of inflammatory cells begin as early as day 3, peaking at day 10, but do not alter morphology of viable tumor on day 6; and (c) the extent of infiltration does not significantly affect tumor size up to and through day 6.

Stenback, et al (31) carried out ultrastructural and functional analyses on 16 freshly biopsied human tumors, 2 mammary and 10 ovarian adenocarcinomas, 2 squamous cell carcinomas, one chondrosarcoma of the bone, 2 transplantation established human ovarian adenocarcinomas and 2 primary rat mammary tumors which were implanted under the renal capsule of 510 normal immunocompetent mice and 180 rats. The results showed successful transplantations of all types of tumors in both animal species. Morphological analysis revealed preserved glandular structures with surface microvilli, mucin and CEA production and partially preserved basement membranes. Treatment with cyclophosphamide, vinblastine, adriamycin and cisplatin caused cell shrinkage, degradation and partial or total disappearence of the tumor cells. Vascularization was distinct in all specimens, and a cellular infiltrate was found frequently but not consistently. A common end stage of the treated xenograft was a fibrotic scar with no cellular activity.

In a recent publication by Cunningham, et al (13) the authors concluded that the 6-day SRCA is of no value with primary surgical explants from gastric cancer because of the host cellular infiltrate evident in untreated control xenografts on day 6 as compared to treated xenografts. They claimed a significantly positive correlation between an inflammation score and increase in size of the xenografts. Unfortunately, this publication is a "Short Communication" and no supportive data correlating score and change in xenograft size is provided. Furthermore, no attempt was made to correlate changes in xenograft size with clinical responses or response rates.

Of particular interest, the authors state that in one assay, instead of treating one of the groups, animals were sacrificed on days 1, 3 and 5 and tumors were examined histologically. They reported a progressive increase in the amount of lymphocytic infiltrate over the period of the assay, but there was also no tumor seen in the transplanted tissues from day 1 despite the presence of abundant tumor in the tissue examined histologically just before transplantation. An observation of this nature raises a question concerning the quality of tissue selected for implantation and the procedure for sectioning $1.0mm^3$ grafts. That fresh surgical explants of gastric cancers will grow when implanted subcapsularly has just recently been reported by Yamauchi et al (19), illustrating the innate growth potential of gastric cancers. Furthermore, they found that correlation between the response of these human tumors to chemotherapy in patients and in 10 or 12-day SRCA's using athymic nudes to be 78.6%

The results of the studies by Aamdal (1, 2), Levi (21), Price (unpublished), Reale (26) and Stenback (31), discussed above, are an unequivical demonstration that human tumor xenografts will grow for at least 4 days when implanted under the renal capsule providing, of course, that uncontaminated, viable tumor tissue is implanted.

SPECIFICITY OF TUMOR RESPONSE IN THE 6-DAY SRC ASSAY AS ILLUSTRATED BY BILATERAL SUBRENAL CAPSULE IMPLANTS

Active drugs reduce the size of a subcapsular tumor xenograft with the degree of tumor sensitivity being reflected by the degree of tumor reression. A drug resistant tumor, on the other hand, experiencing no oncolytic effects exhibits either no change, or an increase in size. Such specificity of tumor response in the 6-day assay period can be easily demonstrated by implanting one kidney with a drug resistant tumor and the contralateral kidney with a drug-sensitive tumor.

Figure 2 illustrates the divergent responses of two transplantable human tumors of different histologic types, an ovarian tumor 207 which was implanted into the right kidney and a melanoma 255 which was implanted into the left kidney. Both tumors in the one group retained as the vehicle treated control showed a +ΔTS. The ovarian tumor responded to cyclophosphamide whereas the melanoma in the contralateral kidney did not. Both tumors responded to dacarbazine. Growth of the ovarian tumor was inhibited by hexamethylmelamine, but the melanoma in the contralateral kidney was relatively resistant.

Such specificity of tumor response is also evident with bilateral xenografts of fresh

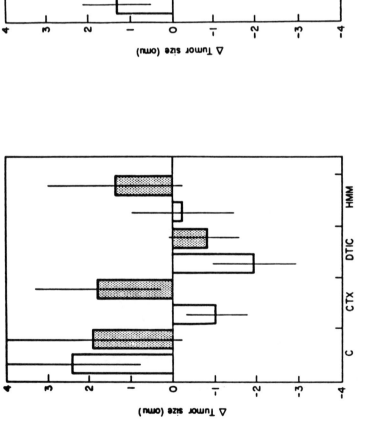

Figure 2. Responses to chemotherapy of bi-lateral subcapsular xenografts of transplantation established human tumors in the 6-Day SRCA: □, MR1-H-207, ovarian, right; ■, MR1-H-255, melanoma, left.

Figure 3. Responses to chemotherapy of bi-lateral subcapsular xenografts of fresh surgical explants (human tumors) in the 6-Day SRCA: □, MR1-H-1291, met. ca., unknown primary, right; ■, MR1-H-382B, ovarian left.

surgical specimens. In Figure 3, a metastatic carcinoma of an unknown primary was implanted into the right kidney and an ovarian carcinoma in the left. Both control tumors produced a +ΔTS. Note the relative sensitivity to adriamycin and cyclophosphamide. The metastatic carcinoma is slightly responsive to 5-FU whereas the ovarian tumor is resistant.

That the evident specificity of tumor response is not the result of the implant site, i.e., whether implanted into the right as contrasted to the left kidney, is indicated by Figure 4. In this study two lines of the M5076 murine ovarian tumor syngeneic with C57BL/6 mice were implanted bilaterally into histocompatible B6C3F$_1$ hybrids. The hexamethylmelamine resistant line was implanted into the left kidney and the sensitive line in the right kidney. The relative drug sensitivity of the two lines is evident in the dose response. Data such as this support the conclusion that the SRC assay is measuring a biological property of the tumor rather than a nonspecific host effect.

HOW WELL DOES THE 6-DAY SRCA PREDICT CLINICAL RESPONSE RATES OF KNOWN ACTIVE CHEMOTHERAPY AGENTS?

If an assay is capable of detecting the drug sensitivities of individual tumors, it should also be able to duplicate clinical response rates when used to screen cancer patient populations for sensitivity to known, clinically active, chemo-therapeutic agents.

In the following example from our own laboratory (9), fresh surgical explants were obtained from 130 human breast tumors and treated in the 6-day SRCA with six clinically active drugs, i.e., drugs known to induce regression of tumors in more than 20% of breast cancer patients. Table 12 compares the response rates obtained with the six drugs in the 6-day SRCA, based upon 130 patients with the response rates obtained

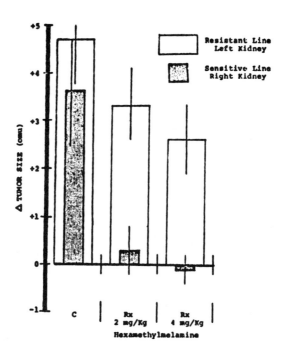

Figure 4. Response of bilaterally implanted
hexamethylmelamine sensitive and resistant
sublines of the transplantable murine M5076
tumor to hexamethylmelamine treatment in
histocompatible mice. ☐ , resistant line
left kidney; ■ , sensitive line right kidney
(Means ± SD).

clinically, based upon 3960 patients, as reported by Carter (11). Most of the patients in the clinical compilation had extensive therapy with endocrine maneuvers or other drugs prior to the single agent therapy, whereas over 93% of the breast tumors tested in the assay were from previously untreated patients. This difference in patient population may account for the somewhat higher response rates for L-PAM, CTX and VCR in the SRCA. Had these six drugs been developmental agents of unknown activity which were being tested for the first time against such a sample of randomly selected human breast tumors, the results not only would have predicted their clinical activity, but also would have provided an indication of the relative potential of each drug for the specific treatment of breast cancer. It is important to point out that from the pattern of tumor responses obtained with this panel of six agents that no single agent was active against all tumors, nor were tumors which were responsive to one agent necessarily responsive to another. The data in this study support the rationale that increasing, not only the number of agents but the number of effective agents in a treatment combination increases the chances of a "therapeutic hit". Of particular importance was the number of tumors responsive to only one or two drugs of a projected three drug combination, such as CMF. One wonders, synergistic activities aside, whether combination chemotherapy would be enhanced for the individual cancer patient if the one or two drugs indicated to be inactive were deleted from a proposed combination in favor of increasing the dose level of the one or two agents with indicated activity.

In an attempt to adapt a predictive in vivo model for head and neck cancers that had clinical relevance and could be performed readily at minimal expense, McCormick et al (24), at the University of Iowa Hospitals and Clinics, utilized the 6-day SRCA to determine chemotherapeutic sensitivities of metastatic primary or recurrent head and neck cancers. Twenty-four tumors from 21

TABLE 12

COMPARISON OF RESPONSE RATES IN THE SUBRENAL CAPSULE ASSAY TO

SINGLE AGENT CHEMOTHERAPY IN PUBLISHED CLINICAL TRIALS:

BREAST CANCERS

Agent	% Response Rate	
	Clinical Experience[1]	SRC Assay[2]
L-PAM	22	42
CTX	34	43
MTX	34	34
5-FU	26	34
VCR	21	32
ADR	35	26

[1] Modified from Henderson and Canellos, New England J. Med. 302: 78-90, 1980. (3960 patients with extensive prior therapy).

[2] Bogden et al. Breast Cancer Research and Treatment 3: 33-38. 1983. (130 patients primarily untreated).

patients were tested. All tests were evaluable. There were 20 squamous cell carcinomas, two melanomas, one adenoid cystic carcinoma and one mucoepidermoid carcinoma. Fourteen of 20 specimens or 70% of squamous cell carcinomas showed statistically significant susceptibility to the oncolytic activity of one or more cytotoxic agents. Although assays of two melanomas indicated susceptibility to several drugs, both the adenoid cystic carcinoma and mucoepidermoid carcinoma were resistant.

In Table 13, the responses of squamous cell tumors in the 6-day SRCA are compared with the clinical responses reported for single agent chemotherapy for these tumors. Despite the difference in the numbers of patients and tumors tested, similar patterns emerge. Each of the four major drugs tested, methotrexate, cyclophosphamide, cisplatin and bleomycin are ranked similarly in both clinical and murine studies. Although too few tumors were tested in the assay to ascertain exact response rates, the response rates obtained by the assay estimated the relative ranking of clinical drug effectiveness.

In assessing the practicability of utilizing the 6-day SRCA as a predictive test system for directing chemotherapy of melanomas, Dumont et al (14), at the Clinic Henry Tagnon, Institut Jules Bordet, Brussels, and the Netherlands Cancer Institute, examined the sensitivity of 24 malignant melanomas to six chemotherapeutic agents. Good correlations were obtained between the percentage of responses in the 6-day SRCA and that of clinical responses for the same drugs (Table 11). The evaluable assay rate was 95%. The response profile provided by the 24 melanomas indicated that drug sensitivity was not all-or-none; one tumor can be sensitive to some drugs and insensitive or resistant to others.

Juhani Maenpaa, et al (22), from the Department of Obstetrics and Gynecology, University of Turku and the Farmos Group Research

TABLE 13

COMPARISON OF RESPONSE RATES IN THE SUBRENAL CAPSULE ASSAY TO
SINGLE AGENT CHEMOTHERAPY IN PUBLISHED CLINICAL TRAILS:
SQUAMOUS CELL TUMORS OF THE HEAD AND NECK

Agent	Clinical Experience[1]		SRC Assay[2]	
	No. Patients	Response %	No. Patients	Response %
Methotrexate (weekly)	100	50	14	71
Cyclophosphamide	77	36	14	57
Cisplatin	108	33	16	19
Bleomycin Sulfate	298	18	15	13

[1]Adapted from Hong and Bromer, New England J. Med. 308: 75-79, 1983.

[2]K.J. McCormick et al. Archives of Otolaryngology 109: 715-718,
1983. University of Iowa Hospitals and Clinics, Iowa City, Iowa

Center, Finland, examined the responsiveness of ovarian cancer to combination chemotherapy in the 6-day SRCA. Fresh surgical explants were obtained from 42 untreated and 19 previously treated ovarian tumors. Fifty-nine (97%) of the assays were evaluable.

The response rate of this group of ovarian tumors to the three drug combination Adriamycin + Cytoxan + Cisplatin was 89%. The clinical response of advanced ovarian cancer to this three drug combination has been comparable, having a reported range of 63%-93% (20, 30, 29). In a subsequent prospective clinical trial, Maenpaa (23) obtained an overall clinical response rate to Adriamycin + Cytoxan + Cisplatin of 57% (13/23) and with primary untreated ovarian cancer a clinical response rate of 65% (13/20). The clinical and assay response rates are compared in Table 14.

INDIVIDUALIZING CANCER CHEMOTHERAPY: ASSAY/CLINICAL CORRELATIONS

The data reviewed above suggest that the 6-day SRCA is adequately predictive to duplicate clinical response rates to chemotherapeutic agents by sampling cancer patient populations with the assay. The question now to be addressed is just how effective the 6-day SRCA is in directing chemotherapy of the individual cancer patient.

Data from clinical studies by their very nature are slow in accumulating. They generally require the attention and/or cooperation of several medical specialties, consent of the patient projected for study, and extensive as well as objective follow-up. The assay/clinical correlations that follow were obtained from four medical centers, and though available correlations are limited in number (311 patients providing 391 trials), they auger well for the predictive value of the 6-day SRCA in clinical oncology.

SRCA/clinical validation data, based on both

TABLE 14

COMPARISON OF RESPONSE RATES IN THE SUBRENAL CAPSULE ASSAY TO THREE

DRUG COMBINATION CHEMOTHERAPY IN PUBLISHED CLINICAL TRIALS:

OVARIAN CANCERS

	Response Rate	
Drug Combination	Clinical Experience[1]	SRC Assay[2]
Adriamycin + Cytoxan + Cisplatin	63% - 93%	65% - 89%

[1]Honetz, N.: Fortschritte in der Chemoterapie des Ovarialkarzinoms.

Stehman, F.B., Ehrlich, C.E., Einhorn, L.H. et al: Long Term fol-low-up and survival in stage III-IV epitherlial ovarian cancer treated with cis-dichlorodiamine platinum, adriamycin and cyclo-phosphamide (PAC). Proc. Am. Soc. Clin. Oncol. 2: 147, 1983.

Schulz, B.O. Hof, K., Friedrich, H-J et al: Experience with combi-nations of cytostatics containing platinum in the treatment of ad-vanced gynaecological carcinomas (Ger.) Geburtsh u Frauenheilk 44: 34, 1984.

[2]Modified from Maenpaa, J., Kangas, L. and Gronroos, M. Department of Obstetrics and Gynaecology, University of Turku and the Farmos Group Research Center, Finland. J. Obstetrics and Gynaecology, 66: 708-713, 1985.

Maenpaa, J. Department of Obstetrics and Gynaecology, University of Turku, Finland. J. Obstetrics and Gynaecology, 66: 715-718, 1985.

retrospective as well as prospective studies, were
obtained from the University of Massachusetts
Medical Center in Worcester, Massachuetts and from
affiliated oncologists comprising the Central
Massachusetts Oncology Group; from the Institut J.
Paoli I. Calmettes in Marseille, France; from the
University of California, Irvine Medical Center in
Orange, California; and from the Department of
Obstetrics and Gynecology, University of Turku,
Finland.

The evaluable assay rates obtained at these
institutions and the responsible investigators are
shown in Table 15. For malignancies of various
histologic types, the overall evaluable assay rate
obtained was 90%. The criteria for an evaluable
assay was similar at all four institutions.

Sensitivity, specificity, efficiency and
predictive value define a laboratory test's
diagnostic accuracy (18). The ability of the
assay to correctly identify clinical responders
(i.e., the sensitivity) and clinical failures
(i.e., the specificity), and its overall ability
to predict the clinical outcome of chemotherapy
(i.e., the efficiency) are described for both
retrospective and prospective clinical trials.

Sensitivity, specificity and efficiency are
intrinsic to the assay, whereas the predictive
value is also markedly affected by the prevalence
of potential responders as well as the prevalence
of potential clinical failures (non-responders) in
a cancer patient population. The positive
predictive value of the assay indicates the
frequency of clinical responders in a patient
population whose tumor is responsive to chemotherapy as indicated by the assay, and the
negative predictive value indicates the frequency
of clinical failures in a patient population whose
tumor is resistant to chemotherapy in the assay
(Table 16).

TABLE 15

EVALUABLE ASSAY RATES IN CLINICAL STUDIES

Investigator and Institution	Type of Malignancies	No. of Patients	Evaluable Assay Rate
R. Favre, et al, Inst. J. Paoli I. Calmettes, Marseille, France	Various	80	88%
T. Griffin, et al, Univ. Mass Medical Center, Worcester	Various	1000	86%
J. Stratton, et al, Univ. Californial Medical Center at Irvine	Gynecologic	242	89%
J. Maenpaa, Univ. of Turku, Turku, Finland	Gynecologic	61	97%

TABLE 16

PARAMETERS OF DIAGNOSTIC ACCURACY* AS APPLIED

TO THE SUBRENAL CAPSULE ASSAY

Parameter	Definition	Formula
SRCA — Potential Patient Response		
Sensitivity	Frequency of correctly identifying clinical responders	TP/TP+FN
Specificity	Frequency of correctly identifying clinical resistance	TN/TN+FP
Efficiency	Frequency of correctly predicting clinical outcome.	TP+TN/ TP+FP+TN+FN
Pos. Predictive Value	Indicates the frequency of clinical responders in patients whose tumor is responsive in the assay.	TP/TP+FP
Neg. Predictive Value	Indicates the frequency of clinical failures in patients whose tumor is non-responsive in the assay.	TN/TN+FN

*Galen, R.S. Statistics, in Gradwohl's Clinical Laboratory Methods and Diagnosis. A.C. Sonnenwirth and L. Jarrett (Eds.), Mosby, St. Louis, 1980, pp. 41-68.

TP = true positive   FP = false positive

TN = true negative   FN = false negative

RETROSPECTIVE CLINICAL STUDIES

In retrospective studies, the patient is treated without benefit of the assay. The decision to treat the patient with specific chemotherapeutic agents is made before the test is run. Drugs for SRCA testing are selected post facto. In such trials, Stratton (32), testing gynecologic tumors, was able to correctly identify 12/18 responders and 58/82 failures for an overall efficiency of 70% (Table 17). Griffin (19), testing tumors of varied histologies, correctly identified 37/38 responders and 16/24 non-responders for an overall efficiency of 85%. Favre (17), also testing malignancies of various histologies correctly identified 8/8 responders and 45/48 non-responders for an overall efficience of 96% with no false negatives. In very limited clinical trials, testing various malignancies, Bogden and Von Hoff (10) obtained a sensitivity of 100% (3/3), a specificity of 80% (16/20), for an overall efficiency of 83% (Table 17).

The activity cut-off points used in the SRCA's by these investigators are also indicated in Table 17. For Stratton, the tumor was a responder if the mean ΔTS (change in tumor size) was negative and significantly different from the saline treated control. The activity criterion used by Griffin was a ΔTS < -1.0 omu cutoff for drug activity. The most stringent criterion was used by Favre, a ΔTS < -1.0 omu that also had to be significantly different from the control (Student "t" test).

In view of the relatively low overall efficiency obtained by Stratton's group, it is important to note the condition and response of the patient population tested and the stringent criteria of clinical tumor response and regression that were applied in the assessment of the response to chemotherapy. A complete response was the absence of all disease at the second look laporatomy. A partial response was a 50% or greater decrease in tumor size at second look laparotomy. Complete clinical resolution of malignant effusion or ascites, tumor hormone

TABLE 17

PREDICTIVE CORRELATIONS BETWEEN SUBRENAL CAPSULE ASSAYS AND CLINICAL RESPONSES

Reference	Clinical Trials	No. Patients	No. Trials	Parameters of Diagnostic Accuracy (%)		
				Sensitivity[1]	Specificity[2]	Efficiency[3]
Stratton, et al (1984)	Retrospective	69	100	12/18 (67%)	58/82 (71%)	70%
	Prospective	66	83	17/20 (85%)	36/63 (57%)	64%
Favre, et al (1986)	Retrospective	80	56	8/8 (100%)	45/48 (84%)	96%
	Prospective		43	19/20 (95%)	26/30 (87%)	90%
Griffin, et al (1983)	Retrospective	55	62	37/38 (97%)	16/24 (67%)	85%
Bogden & Von Hoff	Retrospective	17	23	3/3 (100%)	16/20 (80%)	83%
Maenpaa (1985)	Prospective	24	24	14/14 (100%)	5/10 (50%)	79%
		311	391	110/121 (91%)	202/277 (73%)	78%

Activity Cut-off Points: Stratton, any $-\Delta TS^*$
Griffin, $\Delta TS < -0.5^*$
Favre, $\Delta TS < -1.0^*$
Bogden and Von Hoff, $\Delta TS < -1.0$

* $\overline{m}$ ΔTS significantly different from control (Student "t" test)

marker titers which returned to normal levels for at least four months, and a palpable mass which decreased 50% or more for at least four months, were also deemed to be partial responses. Patients with these responses were categorized as sensitive to the chemotherapy. All other responses were categorized as resistant to the chemotherapy. There were 24 patients who failed the chemotherapy which the SRCA predicted their tumors should have responded to; eight of these patients had been off the therapy for 1-12 months before progession (mean 5.3 months, median 5.0 months), seven had non-measurable residual disease and had no evidence of disease until the second look surgery, and seven had massive residual disease at the initiation of the chemotherapy. Mean time interval for second look surgery was 9.5 months.

PROSPECTIVE CLINICAL STUDIES

To determine how effectively an assay can select chemotherapeutic agents for treatment of the individual cancer paitent, one must complete the assay and make the prediction of activity prior to initiation of therapy. Treatment of the patient on the basis of assay results is not necessary as long as the drug being administered has been tested in the assay.

In the following assay/clinical correlations, SRCA's were performed before the patients received chemotherapy and the drugs for testing were selected on the basis of what the patient was likely to receive, a decision made by the treating physician without knowledge of assay results Thus, the assay was used prospectively to predict clinical sensitivity or resistance.

In the study of gynecologic tumors, primarily ovarian, by Stratton et al (32), approximately half of the patients that were evaluated prospectively had fialed first line chemotherapy and most of the tumors were well advanced. Table 17 illustrates the correlation of the clinical

response of the patient to the administered
chemotherapy with the response predicted by the
SRCA. Of the 83 possible correlations, there were
17 true positives (S/S), 27 false positives (R/S),
36 true negatives (R/R), and only three false
negatives (R/S). These data indicate that the
sensitivity of the assay is 85%, the specificity
is 57%, and the overall efficiency is 64%.

In examining the relatively low specificity
which is caused by false positives (9) in the
assay, it is important to point out that of the 27
false positives, 10 were on tumors from patients
who had had a previous chemotherapy to which seven
failed and three only partially responded. Of the
false positive patients, 14 had large residual
disease at the initiation of chemotherapy.
Following chemotherapy, seven of the false
positive patients had non-measurable residual
disease with no evidence of disease until the
second-look surgery, seven had stable disease for
4-8 months before progession, and one had stable
disease and was off chemotherapy for four months
before disease progression. Interestingly, five
of the false positive tumors were from patients
whose tumor specimens tested as resistant to the
same chemotherapy at the second-look surgery.

Of the thirty-one prospective analysis
patients that had prior chemotherapy, only two
responded to the new chemotherapy. The SRCA
predicted one of these responses. In this previously treated and relapsed group there were 34
clinical failures of 41 drug trials. The SRCA
predicted 24 of these failures.

It should be emphasized that most of the
positive clinical correlates (true positives) in
the study overall were from patients who had
surgically proven disease regression. In most
cases, surgery was 10 months after the initiation
of chemotherapy. The mean time interval was 9.5
months and the shortest interval was six months.
Only one of the positive clinical correlates was
less than six months and that was a 4-month

partial response in a suboptimally resected patient.

Prevalence of responders in a clinical setting indicates the frequency of potential responders where the optimum chemotherapy is known a priori. The frequency of positive test results in responding patients (sensitivity) and the frequency of negative test results in non-responding patients (specificity) are independent of prevalence of the potential for clinical response. However, the predictive value of an assay is very dependent on the prevlance of potential responders. Prevalence of clinical response to chemotherapy in the prospective patients studied by Stratton, et al, was 20.5% (total number of responders over number tested). If the SRCA were no more predictive than chance, the sensitivity plus the specificity would be equal to 100% and the predictive value would be equal to the prevalence of response (20%). Neither of these is true, sensitivity plus specificity was 142%, the positive predictive value was 39%, and the negative predictive value was 92%.

Before the SRCA results are known the patient belongs in a population with a probability of response to chemotherapy equal to the prevalence. The prevalence of response of the prospective group was 20.5%, that is, 20.5% of the treated patients responded to the chemotherapy. After the SRCA results are known, the patient belongs in a population with a probability of response equal to the predictive value of the positive test results, in this case 39%. If the SRC assay were no better than chance, predictive value would be equal to prevalence. Thus, the positive predictive accuracy with the SRCA was 1.9-fold better than chance alone. The prospective patients who had failed the previous chemotherapy, had a prevalence of response of 4.9%. The SRCA improved the probability to 9.1% also an increase of 1.9-fold. Stratton points out that on the basis of her results, and considering the class of patients studied in her prospective correlations, the probability of a clinical response <u>without</u> the assay was 20.5%. The probability of clinical response if it were <u>assay directed</u> was 39.6%.

In the prospective clinical studies being carried out at the Institut J. Paoli I. Calmettes, Favre <u>et al</u> (17) systematically looked for SRCA/clinical response correlations utilizing UICC clinical response criteria applied to advanced cancers of the head and neck, breast, colorectal, endometrium, testis, ovary, lymphomas, a bone sarcoma and a metastatic adenocarcinoma. Change in tumor size was based upon the product of two diameters rather than the sum of two diameters as used by Bogden <u>et al</u> (6). Table 17 summarizes the SRCA/clinical response correlations obtained by Favre and his group in the prospective study. A total of 43 assay/clinical correlations were possible. Of 20 clinically sensitive responses, the assay accurately predicted 19 or 95%. Of the 30 clinically resistant responses, the assay accurately predicted 26 or 87%. Thus, the overall predictive accuracy of the SRCA in Favre's experience was 90%. Of particular importance, stimulation of tumor growth was observed in the SRCA in two cases, one of which was clinically correlated.

In view of the relatively high evaluable assay rate (97%), and the excellent correlation of assay/clinical response rates obtained with drug combinations in ovarian cancers (22), Maenpaa evaluated the ability of the assay to <u>predict prospectively</u> the response of advanced ovarian cancer to combination chemotherapy (23).

Of 52 ovarian cancer patients providing tissues for SRCA, there were 24 patients with advanced or recurrent disease in whom the results of the SRCA and the clinical response to combination chemotherapy could be compared on a prospective basis. All 24 patients included in this prospective study had disseminated disease and none had been operated radically so that drug effects could be reliably evaluated. Clinical responses were evaluated as recommended by the Meeting on Standardization of Reporting of Results of Cancer Treatment for non-measurable, evaluable disease (25).

Treatment of 20 of the 24 patients followed a national program, according to which they received a combination of ADR, CTX and Cisplatin. Samples for SRCA were obtained at primary laparotomy before any other treatment and in each assay ADR + CTX + Cisplatin was one of the drug combinations tested. Thus, a prospective correlative design (27) rather than randomization was used in most cases.

The clinical response was evaluated every four weeks before each new course of therapy. After therapy, the patients were followed up at two to three month intervals. Responses were confirmed by computerized tomography and ultra-sonography. Of the remaining four patients, three had a recurrent disease and one had breast cancer metastases to the ovaries and' peritoneal surfaces.

There were 14/24 (58%) patients who responded objectively (CR+PR) to the multidrug therapy used. The over-all response rate to ADR + CTX + Cisplatin was 57% (13/23) and of primary untreated ovarian cancer 65% (13/20). According to the 3-grade interpretation of SRCA sensitivity criteria used, 8/14 (57%) of these tumors were sensitive, 6/14 (43%) were intermediately sensitive and none were resistant in the SRCA. The median duration of response was 10.5+ months for the patients with tumors graded as sensitive and 8+ months for those with intermediate sensitive tumors. Twelve patients were relaparotomized and samples for the SRCA were taken at relaparotomy in eight instances. Seven of these repeat assays were evaluable. Four tumors were clearly less sensitive to ADR + CTX + Cisplatin after five to ten courses of therapy than before treatment, and the disease progressed shortly after the second-look operation in spite of chemotherapy. The sensitivity of two tumors had decreased slightly but remained in the same range. One patient is disease-free at 17 months after the primary operation, while another patient relapsed two months after relaparotomy. The sensitivity of one tumor had remained unchanged. This patient relapsed only 17 months after relaparotomy.

Using a 3-grade interpretation of drug response in the assay (sensitive, intermediately sensitive and resistant), an efficiency of 79% was achieved (Table 17). All objective clinical responses (14/14) were predicted by the assay with no false negatives yielding a sensitivity of 100%. There were, however, five false positives. Importantly, the SRCA was able to detect the development of drug resistance. In the small series of repeat measurements of drug activity, 4/7 assays showed a marked weakening of drug response after therapy, and the disease progressed thereafter.

An even more stringent evaluation of a predictive quality is a clinical study in which the patient is treated with the chemotherapeutic agent indicated as most active in the assay. The assay selects the drug for treatment, not the physician.

On the basis of the promising results obtained in the retrospective analysis of the SRCA/clinical correlations, Griffin et al (19) initiated the following prospective, decision aiding, trials. All patients involved in this study had advanced metastatic disease. In this study patients were treated in a prospective fashion wth the single agent producing the greatest amount of growth inhibition or regression in the SRCA. Chemotherapy was administered according to standard dosages and schedules. Patient eligibility requirements for protocol entry were: metastatic malignancy for which there is no standard therapy of clinical value, or which has become refractory to conventional therapy; an evaluable SRCA; a reproducible, objective measurement of disease; performance status of three or better, expected duration of survival of at least eight weeks; and a signed informed consent to an experimental study.

Patients showing stable disease, or partial response, after two cycles of therapy were continued on single agent chemotherapy, or alternately switched to combination chemotherapy including the original agent and a second active agent, at the discretion of their attending physician. Patients showing progressive disease after one complete cycle of therapy were considered treatment failures and were withdrawn from the protocol. Standard definitions of response evaluation were employed (25).

Forty-seven patients with chemotherapy refractory cancers were entered on the prospective study. Fourteen histologic types of malignancies were represented. These 47 patients provided 50 clinical trials. Ten clinical trials were judged unevaluable for response due to reasons such as early death, lost to follow-up, entered with no measurable disease, or early withdrawal due to drug toxicity. Therefore, 37 patients and 40 clinical trials were available for response evaluation. All responses required the standard criteria for partial response, complete response, and progressive disease. Files of responding patients were reviewed by the chief clinical investigators in association with clinicians caring for the patients.

Of the clinically evaluable group, 14 of 37 patients (38%) and 14 of 70 clinical courses (42%) showed partial or complete response. The median duration of response in all patients was four months. These response rates are of particular interest because the prevalence of response to chemotherapy in this class of heavily pretreated patients is, at best, 20%. It is of interest to note that both the prevalence of responders in this patient population, where the results of the SRCA are known, and the positive predictive accuracy of the SRCA in this study are identical to those reported by Stratton, et al (32).

Importantly, the probability of patient response showed a strong relationship to single agent drug activity in the assay (Table 18). For the small group of patints with 60% tumor fragment regression by day 6 ($\geq$3.0 omu change in tumor size), six of seven patients responded (86%). Moreover, the duration of tumor response seemed clearly related to single agent drug activity in the assay. Responses in the group with <0.3 omu single agent activity were short-lived (median duration of remission, six weeks) in contrast to patients with greater degree of regression in the assay (median duration of remission, eight months). Patients in the latter group also demonstrated significantly increased survival as compared to non-responders to chemotherapy.

Transplanted human tumor xenografts in nude mice maintain chemotherapy sensitivity profiles, to a great extent, over serial passage. The concordance of drug activity in serial biopsy specimens in the same patient was similarly determined. In this study, drug activity for tumor specimens from the same patient, obtained more than four weeks apart, was analyzed in both treated and untreated patients (Table 19). Twenty-four patients had serial biopsies of their tumors performed, with the same drugs screened against the initial and subsequent biopsy specimens. Sixteen patients had no intervening chemotherapy; however, eight of these 16 patients had intervening radiotherapy, and two had intervening hormonal therapy. These 16 patients provided 107 serial drug trials for analysis. Of 71 drugs active in the first assay, 47 (66%) were active in the repeat assay. Of 31 drugs inactive in the first assay, 25 were inactive in the second assay. This relationship between activity of a given drug in the first and subsequent assays, despite the complexities of the clinical situation, is highly significant (p < 0.0001, Fischer Exact Test) and suggests that the assay is identifying an intrinsic biological property of

TABLE 18

CLINICAL RESPONE RATES AND DURATION OF RESPONDSES

IN RELATION TO TUMOR REGRESSION IN ASSAY

(Prospective - Decision Aiding Trials)

Tumor Regression In SRC Assay	Clinical Response Rate*		Median Duration of Responses
≥ 3.0 omu	6/7	86%	8 months
≤ 2.9 omu	8/30	27%	6 weeks
All Regression:	14/37	38%	4 months

*7/37 (19%) patient population highly responsive in assay.

TABLE 19

CONCORDANCE OF DRUG ACTIVITY IN SERIAL BIOPSIES

. 16 Patients with no intervening chemotherapy

⎡ 8 with intervening radiotherapy ⎤
⎣ 2 with intervening hormonal therapy ⎦

. 107 serial drug trials for analysis

Drug Activity	Concordance*	
Of 71 drugs active in first assay, 41 drugs active in repeat assay.	47/71	66%
Of 31 drugs inactive in first assay, 25 drugs inactive in repeat assay.	25/31	81%
Overall concordance with no intervening chemotherapy.	72/102	72%

* p <0.0001 Fisher Exact Test

the tumor.

In contrast, in ten patients with intervening chemotherapy, drugs active in the first assay were active in only 25% of repeat assays, suggesting the emergence of drug resistance. Nine of these ten patients showed assay resistance to one or more of the chemotherapeutic agents they had received in the inter-assay period.

Additional retrospective and prospective assay/clinical correlations are desirable. Nonetheless, the data from both the retrospective and prospective clinical studies carried out in several reputable medical institutions, suggest that chemotherapy of the individual cancer patient's can be effectively improved by pretesting the patient's tumor against a battery of therapeutic agents in the 6-day SRCA.

EMERGENCE OF DRUG RESISTANCE FOLLOWING EFFECTIVE CHEMOTHERAPY: ASSAY/CLINICAL RESULTS

Disease progression following an initial favorable response, despite continuing chemotherapy, is the clinical manifestation of the emergence of drug resistance. Whether this clinical phenomenon reflects the initial sensitivity and elimination of a major tumor cell population, which then permits the emergence of minor drug resistant populations, or the induction of resistance in originally sensitive populations, is of little comfort to the relapsing patient.

The problem of pleiotropic cross resistance is also a clinical reality. Whether to continue chemotherapy and with which drug(s) in the face of disease progression is certainly relevant, not only to the oncologist but to the survival and quality of life of the relapsing patient.

The objective of this section is to provide examples wherein sequential SRCA's on tumor samples taken before and after effective chemotherapy clearly indicated not only the emergence of drug resistance but the ability to detect effective new agents in the face of stable disease.

Table 20 illustrates the responses of sequential biopsies of an oesophageal carcinoma taken approximately five months apart and tested in the SRCA. Of the seven drugs tested against the initial biopsy specimen, three met activity criteria. The patient was subsequently treated with the two drugs indicated to be most active in the assay, i.e., vincristine and 5-fluorouracil and showed a good objective clinical response. Assay results of the second biopsy indicated the tumor to be unresponsive to all drugs tested including the two previously active agents with which the patient had been treated in the interim.

Table 21 illustrates the responses of a squamous cell carcinoma in sequential assays run approximately nine months apart. Of the seven drugs tested against the initial biopsy specimen, five met activity criteria. The patient was treated with the single most active agent as indicated by the assay, i.e., methotrexate, with a good clinical response. The second biopsy specimen was resistant to all drugs tested including methotrexate, cisplatin and cyclophosph- amide, which had been active prior to treatment.

Table 22 summarizes the sequential assays and clinial responses of a malignant lymphoma. This patient was of particular interest having been admitted as a candidate for palliative care with a very poor prognosis and a clinical history extending over seven years of intensive chemo- therapy with remissions and relapses. The first assay indicated bleomycin and adriamycin to be most active. Treatment with these agents induced a good clinical response. With stabilization of remission, another biopsy was taken and tested against bleomycin and adriamycin as well as five new agents. Of the seven agents tested, bleomycin nd adriamycin now ranked last in order of activity and dacarbazine and prednisone ranked as most

TABLE 20

DRUG RESISTANCE FOLLOWING EFFECTIVE CHEMOTHERAPY

TUMOR: POORLY DIFFERENTIATED OESOPHAGEAL CARCINOMA

MRI-H-329A 13 April 1981			MRI-H-329B 1 September 1981	
Drug	ΔTS (omu)		Drug	ΔTS (omu)
VCR	-3.5		F-FU	-0.1
5-FU	-2.3		CTX	0
CCNU	-2.2	RX	BLEO	0
cis-DDP	-1.0	(VCR + 5-FU)	DHAD	+0.3
CTX	-0.5	⟶	VCR	+0.3
ADR	-0.4	Good Response	BAN-HCl	+0.6
MTX	-0.3		ADR	+0.9
Control	+1.6		Control	+0.4

Tumor Responsive: ΔTS < -1.0 omu

VCR, vincristine; 5-FU, 5-Fluorouracil; CCNU, lomustine; cis-
DDP, cis-platinum; CTX, cyclophosphamide; ADR, adriamycin; MTX,
methotrexate; BLEO, bleomycin; DHAD, mitoxantrone; BAN-HCl,
bisantrene hydrochloride.

TABLE 21

DRUG RESISTANCE FOLLOWING EFFECTIVE CHEMOTHERAPY

TUMOR: SQUAMOUS CELL CARCINOMA, METASTATIC, PRIMARY (?)

MRI-H-309A 21 November 1981			MRI-H-309B 1 September 1981	
Drug	ΔTS (omu)		Drug	ΔTS (omu)
MTX	-4.0		cis-DDP	+0.5
CTX	-3.0		BLEO	+0.7
5-FU	-1.6	RX	MTX	+0.7
cis-DDP	-1.3	(MTX)	ARA-C	+0.8
ADR	-1.1	⟶	CTX	+0.9
VCR	+0.5	Good Response	AND	+1.3
CCNU	+0.5		BAN-HCl	+1.6
Control	+0.4		Control	+1.7

Tumor Responsive: ΔTS < -1.0 omu

MTX, methotrexate; CTX, cyclophosphamide; 5-FU, 5-Fluorouracil;
cis-DDP, cis-platinum; ADR, adriamycin; VCR, vincristine, CCNU,
lomustine; BLEO, bleomycin; ARA-C, cytosine arabinoside; AND,
anthracenedione; BAN-HCl, bisantrene hydrochloride.

TABLE 22

DRUG RESISTANCE FOLLOWING EFFECTIVE CHEMOTHERAPY

TUMOR: MALIGNANT LYMPHOMA

MRI-H-309A 22 December 1981			MRI-H-309B 25 February 1981		
Drug	ΔTS (omu)		Drug	ΔTS (omu)	
BLEO	-3.1		DTIC	-3.4	
ADR	-2.1		PRED	-2.4	
MTX	-1.4		ARA-C	-1.9	
CTX	-1.0	Rx (BLEO + ADR)	ACT-D	-1.8	Rx (DTIC + PRED)
VBL	-0.8	⟶	VCR	-1.3	⟶
cis-DDP	+0.4	Good Response	BLEO	-1.2	Good Response
			ADR	-1.0	
Control	+0.3		Control	-0.5	

Tumor Responsive: ΔTS < -1.0 omu

BLEO, bleomycin; ADR, adriamycin; MTX, methotrexate; CTX, cyclophosphamide; VLB, vinblastine; cis-DDP, cis-platinum; DTIC, de-
carbazine; PRED, prednisone; ARA-C, cytosine arabinoside; ACT-D,
actinoside; ACT-D, actinomycin D; VCR, vincristine.

active. Treated with the two active agents, an almost complete remission was obtained.

Emergence of a drug resistance in the assay reflects the phenomenon of drug resistance observed clinically. That the assay can detect the emergence of such resistance suggest that practicability of sequential assays, during a prolonged chemotherapeutic regimen, to more effectively tailor chemotherapy for the individual cancer patient.

PREDICTIVE VALUE OF THE 6-DAY SRCA

Combining the results of all the retrospective and prospective clinical studies, the overall sensitivity of the SRCA is 91%, the specificity is 73%, and the efficiency is 78%. Utilizing these parameters of the SRCA, the positive predictive value of the assay is estimated to be 70% when the prevalence of responders in a cancer patient population is 40%. It is estimated to be 84% when the prevalence of responders in a cancer patient population is 60%. And, it is estimated to be 93% when the prevalence of responders in the patient population is 80%. These data suggest that factors which would increase the prevalence of responders in the patient population of interest, e.g., the evaluation of patients with no previous chemotherapy, or the development of an increasing number of effective chemotherapeutic agents, will result in increasing the positive predictive value of the SRCA.

With an increasing number of "effective" chemotherapeutic agents entering the clinic, it is time that individual patient treatment be guided by considerations more specific and relevant than response rates. Placing the vulnerable cancer patient into Phase I or Phase II clinical trials has been an effective method for evaluating the activity of new agents, but at a terrible price to the unresponsive patient. We are of the same opinion as Weisenthal (34). If investigators were to put forth more effort into using presently

available assay systems appropriately to discover
and test new methods for detecting drug
sensitivity or, alternatively, circumventing drug
resistance in fresh human tumor speciments, then
surprising progress in improving cancer chemotherapy might be achieved. "It is time to stop
quibbling about which approach to chemosensitivity testing is most theoretically pure and
intellectually satisfying and to begin selecting
assay systems for specific applications based upon
their practicability and usefulness for these
specific applications."

Acknowledgement: The authors acknowledge and
thank Lisa Marolda for her patience, perseverence
and skill in preparing a rather lengthy and table
filled manuscript for photo-offset printing.

REFERENCES

1. Aamdal, S., Fodstad, O., Kaalhus, O. and Pihl,
    A. Reduced Antineoplastic Activity in Mice of
    Cisplatin Administered With High Salt Con-
    centration in the Vehicle. J.N.C.I. 73:
    743-752, 1984.

2. Aamdal, S., Fodstad, O. and Pihl, A. Human
    Tumor Xenografts Transplanted Under The Renal
    Capsule of Conventional Mice. Growth Rates
    and Host Immune Response. Int. J. Cancer 34:
    725-730, 1984.

3. Aamdal, S., Fodstad, O., Nesland, J. M. and
    Pihl, A. Characteristics of Human Tumor
    Xenografts Transplanted Under the Renal
    Capsule of Immunocompetent Mice. Br. J. Cancer
    51: 347-356, 1985.

4. Abrams, J., Jacobovitz, D., Dumont, P., Semal, P., Mammen, P., Klastersky, J. and Atassi, G. Subrenal Capsule Assay of Fresh Human Tumors: Problems and Pitfalls. Eur. J. Cancer Clin. Oncol. 22: 1387-1394, 1986.

5. Bennett, J.A., Pilon, V.A. and MacDowell, R.T. Evaluation of Growth and Histology of Human Tumor Xenografts Implanted Under the Renal Capsule of Immunocompetent and Immunodeficient Mice. Cancer Res. 45: 4963-4969, 1985.

6. Bogden, A.E., Kelton, D.E., Cobb, W.R. and Esber, H.J. A rapid screening method for testing chemotherapeutic agents against human tumor xenografts. In: Houchens & Ovejera, Proceedings of the Symposium on The Use of Athymic (Nude) Mice in Cancer Research. New York: Gustav Fischer, 231-250, 1978.

7. Bogden, A. E., Griffin, T. W., Reich, S. D., Contanza, M.E. and Cobb, W.R. Predictive Testing with the Subrenal Capsule Assay Cancer Treat. Rev. 11: 113-124, 1984.

8. Bogden, A.E., Hnatowitch, D.J., Doherty, P.W. and Griffin, T.W. A Method for Estimating In Vivo Localization of Monoclonal Antibody in Surgical Explants of Human Tumors. Proc. Am. Assoc. Cancer Res., 24: 1983.

9. Bogden, A. E., Costanza, M. E., Reich, S. D., Griffin, T.W. and Cobb, W.R. Chemotherapy Responsiveness of Human Breat Tumors in the 6-Day Subrenal Capsule Assay: An Update. Breast Cancer Research and Treatment 3: 33-38, 1983.

10. Bogden, A.E. and Von Hoff, D.D. Comparison of the Human Tumor Cloning and Subrenal Capsule Assay. Cancer Res. 44: 1087-1090, 1984.

11. Carter, S.K. Chemotherapy of Breast Cancer: Current Status In: J.C. Heuson, W.H. Mattheien and M. Rozencweig (Eds.), Breast Cancer:

Trends in Research and Treatment. Raven Press, New York, 1976, pp. 193-215.

12. Cobb, W. R., LePage, D. J., Lohnes, S. and Bogden, A.E. Human Tumor Xenograft Response in the 6-Day Subrenal Capsule Assay (SRCA): A Comparison of Treatment Schedules Proc. A.A.C.R. 27: 383, 1986.

13. Cunningham, D., Jack, A., McMurdo, D. F. S., Soukop, M., McArdle, C.S., Carter, D.C. and Kaye, S.B. The 6-Day Subrenal Capsule Assay is of No Value with Primary Surgical Explants from Gastric Cancer. "Short Cummunication". Br. J. Cancer 54: 519-523, 1986.

14. Dumont, P., van der Esch, E.P., Jabri, M., Lejeune, F. and Atassi, G. Chemosensitivity of Human Melanoma Xenografts in Immuno-competent Mice and Its Histological Evaluation. Int. J. Cancer 33: 447-451, 1984.

15. Edelstein, M.B., Fiebig, H.H., Smink, J., Van Putten, L.M. and Schuchhardt, C. Comparison Between Macroscopic and Microscopic Evaluation of Tumor Responsiveness Using the Subrenal Capsule Assay. Eur. J. Cancer Clin. Oncol. 19: 995-1009, 1983.

16. Edelstein, M. B., Smink, T., Ruiter, D. J., Visser, W. and Van Putten, L.M. Improvements and Limitations of the Subrenal Capsule Assay for Determining Tumor Sensitivity to Cytostatic Drugs. Eur. J. Cancer Clin. Oncol. 20: 1549-1556, 1984.

17. Favre, R., Marotia, L., Drancourt, M., Jaquemier, J., Delpero, J.R., Guerinel, G. and Carcassonne, Y. 6-Day Subrenal Capsule Assay (SRCA) as a Predictor of the Response of Advanced Cancers to Chemotherapy. Eur. J. Cancer Clin. Oncol. 22: 1171-1178, 1986.

18. Galen, R.S. Statistics, in Gradwohl's Clini-cal Laboratory Methods and Diagnosis. A.C.

Sonnewirth and L. Jarrett (Eds.), Mosby, St. Louis, 1980, pp. 41-68.

19. Griffin, T. W., Bogden, A. E., Reich, S. D., Antonelli, D., Hunter, R.E., Ward, A., Yu, D.T., Greene, H.L. and Costanza, M.E. Initial Clinial Trials of the Subrenal Capsule Assay as a Predictive of Tumor Response to Chemotherapy. Cancer 52: 2185-2192. 1981.

20. Honetz, N. Fortschritte in der Chemotherpie de Ovarialkarzinoms. WMW (13/14): 319, 1982

21. Levi, F.A., Blum, J.P., Lemaigre, G., Bourut, C., Reinberg, A. and Mathe, G. A Four-Day Subrenal Capsule Assay for Testing the Effectiveness of Anticancer Drugs Against Human Tumors. Cancer Res. 44: 2260-2667.

22. Maenpaa, J., Kangas, L. and Gronroos, M. Response of Ovarian Cancer to combined Cytotoxic Agents in the Subrenal Capsule Assay. J. Obstetrics and Gynecology, 66: 708-713, 1985.

23. Maenpaa, J. The Subrenal Capsule Assay as Predictor of the Clinical Response of Ovarian Cancer to Combination Chemotherapy. J. Obstetrics and Gynecology, 66: 715-718, 1985.

24. McCormick, K.J., Panje, W.R., Seltzer, S. and Merrick, R.H. Single Agent Chemotherapy for Head and Neck Cancers. The Murine Subrenal Capsule Assay. Archives of Otolaryngology 109: 715-718, 1983.

25. Miller, A. B., Hoogstratten, B., Staguet, M. and Winkler, A. Reporting Results of a Cancer Treatment. Cancer 47: 207-214, 1981.

26. Reale, F., Bogden, A. E., Griffin, T. and Costanza, M. The Preservation of Histologic Morphology of Human Tumor Explants in Subrenal Capsule Assay. Proc. Am. Assoc. Cancer Res., 25: 372, 1984.

27. Salmon, S.E. Clinical Correlation of Drug Sensitivity, Proress in Clinical and Biological Research. Vol. 48, Cloning of Human Tumor Cells. Edited by S.E. Salmon. New York: Alan R. Liss, Inc. 265-285, 1980.

28. Sands, H., Jones., P. L., Neacy, W., Camin, L.L. and Gallagher, B.M. A Comparison of the Ability of Radioiodinated Monoclonal Anti-Rat Thy 1 (0X7) to Image SL2 Tumors Located Subcutaneously or in the Subrenal Capsule. J. Nuc. Med., (Abstract) 24: 102, 1983.

29. Schultz, B.O., Hof, K., Friedrich, H-J. et al: Experiences with combinations of Cytostatics Containing Platinum in the Treatment of Advanced Gynaecological Carcinomas (Ger.). Geburtsch u Franuenheilk 44: 34, 1984.

30. Stehman, F. B., Ehrlich, C. E., Einhorn, L. H. et al: Long Term Follow-Up and Survival in Stage III-IV Epithelial Ovarian Cancer Treated with Cis-dichlorodiamine Platinum, Adriamycin and Cyclophosphamide (PAC). Proc. Am. Soc. Clin. Oncol. 2: 147, 1983.

31. Stenback, Wasenius, V. M., and Kangas, L. Morphology of Transplanted Tumors and Drug Induced Regression In The Subrenal Capsule Assay (SRCA) of Mice and Rats. Ann. Chir. et Gyraecol 74 (Suppl. 199): 31-37, 1985.

32. Stratton, J. A., Kucera, P. R., Micha, J. P., Rettenmaier, M.A., Braly, P.S., Berman, M.L. and Disaia, P.J. The Subrenal Capsule Tumor Implant Assay as a Predictor of Clinical Response to Chemotherapy: Three Years of Experience. Gynecologic Oncology 19: 336-347, 1984.

33. Venditti, J.M. Preclinical Drug Development: Rationale and Methods. Sem. Oncol. 8: 349-361, 1981.

34. Weisenthal, L.M. Clones, Dyes, Nuclides, Mouse Kidneys, and Virions: A New-Clonogenic Assay for Tumor Chemosensitivity. Perspective and Commentaries. Eur. J. Cancer Clin. Oncol. 23: 9-12, 1987.

35. Yamauchi, M., Ichihashi, H., Kondo, T., Yamamoto, K., and Takagi, H. Chemotherapy Responsiveness of Human Gastric Cancer Implanted in Subrenal Capsules of Nude Mice. Proc. Am. Assoc. Cancer Res., 28: 428, 1987.

Prediction of Response to Cancer Therapy, pages 205-212
© 1988 Alan R. Liss, Inc.

SUBRENAL CAPSULE ASSAY (SRCA) IN HUMAN TUMORS

Lauri Kangas, Alexander van Assendelft, Matti
Grönroos, Pähr-Einar Hellström, Hannu Käpylä,
Juhani Mäenpää, Seppo Pyrhönen, Peter Roberts,
Timo Romppanen, Pekka Saarelainen and Lauri Tammi-
lehto

Farmos Group, Research Center, Box 425, 20101 Tur-
ku, Finland (L.K., H.K.), Kontioniemi (A. van A.,
T.R.) and Meltola (P-E.H., P.S.) Hospitals, Clinic
of Obstetrics and Gynecology (M.G., J.M.), Turku
University Central Hospital, IV Surgical Clinic
(P.R.), Radiotherapy Clinic (S.P.), Dept. of Pul-
monary Medicine (L.T.), Helsinki University
Central Hospital, Finland

INTRODUCTION

Subrenal capsule assay is one of the individual predictive tests aimed at individually tailored cancer chemotherapy. It is the only in vivo test used for this purpose.
The principle of individual cancer chemotherapy is really
worth noticing. It offers two main advantages when compared
to classical animal tumor models and statistical selection
of chemotherapy: 1) improved quality of chemotherapy: more
and better responses 2) more effective development of new
drugs. So, the goal is paramount and there should be space
for every investigator working with in vitro or in vivo
predictive assays.

The aim of the present work was to evaluate SRCA in
fresh clinical tumor samples, especially success rate and
concordance of the assay results with the clinical response.
In several samples SRCA and histological evaluation were
compared. Furthermore we wanted to investigate the most
critical steps of SRCA and to evaluate if any improvements
could be made to the original Bogden's method.

The original Bogden's method was used except that in most samples two tumor pieces were transplanted to each animal.

EXPERIENCES OF THE USE OF SRCA IN FRESH TUMOR SAMPLES

The strongest arguments in favour of SRCA are as follows:

1. microarchitecture of the tissue retained
2. most cells are in their original surrounding
3. cells grow throughout the assay
4. high success rate
5. transplantation technically reliable
6. evaluation resembles "real clinical situation"

These advantages of SRCA are strong enough to justify thorough evaluation, i.e. prospective and retrospective clinical studies using SRCA guided chemotherapy. On the other hand some published negative experiences indicate that SRCA has certain critical steps which should be studied before the assay can be recommended as a routine predictive assay.

The strongest arguments presented against SRCA are as follows (Edelstein et al, 1983; Cunningham et al, 1986):

1. 1 mm^3 piece does not represent the whole tumor
2. no tumor cells in the implant
3. immunological rejection impairs tumor size measurement
4. evaluation not reliable

We wish to respond these items in the light of our own experience.

1. A solid tumor is always a mixture of different cell types. The heterogenicity is unavoidable, not only in SRCA but in all in vitro and in vivo assays. The heterogenicity is and will be a problem in all predictive assays. The heterogenicity should be accepted, because it must be accepted clinically, and on the other hand intensive attempts to decrease the heterogenicity gives selected cell populations. The assay with randomly selected cell populations is hardly more reliable than the pieces of tumor.

Another serious point could be the heterogenicity of metastases. We have found in preliminary tests that different metastases may have similar or different response to drug combinations. It would be good to carry out a separate test from individual metastases. This is practically impossible. SRCA from two differently localised metastases might give valuable information of the heterogeneity.

2. In histological evaluations lack of tumor cells in the sample has been clearly documented (Cunningham et al, 1986). Conclusion has been: SRCA is not valid. This conclusion is not necessarily correct, because another conclusion could be: selection of the samples has failed. Selection of the sample for SRCA is of utmost importance. Poor sample means always poor assay. Therefore all procedures which influence selection should be carefully controlled and all participating persons should be informed of the risks of poor sample selection.

a. Surgeon who takes the primary sample: It might be wise to show the surgeons in practice the transplantation procedure to give an impression of how small pieces are needed and how they should be placed in the transportation medium. All surgeons participating the trials have to be informed. Cooperation of surgeon and pathologist is important. However, well trained pathologists are usually not available routinely for sample selection. The surgeon is in critical position.

b. Selection of 1 mm³ pieces for the actual assay is performed in the laboratory. Careful training, preferably together with a pathologist, is necessary. Failed selection completely destroys the assay. Therefore, time should not be saved in this working step. Evidently there are differences in tumor cell content of different tumors. In gynecological cancers we have seldom had any difficulties in getting active tumor tissue into the SRCA pieces. In lung cancer we could not find tumor cells in 10 out of the 32 samples. In addition 7 samples contained only a small fraction of tumor cells. The present ways in sample selection are apparently not optimal. New ideas and systematic research is needed. Vital staining, use of phase contrast microscope, and selecting more pieces for SRCA are some possible approaches which could help the selection. So could also further investigation of the influence of tumor size on the assay; small pieces with high cancer cell density can often be obtained and could be selected in a reliable manner for SRCA under a phase contrast microscope.

3. Immunological rejection or signs of that have been demonstrated in several papers. Bogden considers rejection at 6 days nonessential. In lung cancers we performed a histological study with 32 samples to evaluate the importance of rejection. The results have been presented in table 1.

TABLE 1. Presence of inflammation and infiltration in lung cancer samples evaluated after the assay by histology. Histological evaluation scale: from +++ = marked share of host cells to - = no infiltration and inflammation. Control animals received saline, chemotherapies were as follows: CDP = cyclophosphamide + doxorubicin + cisplatin, DMF = doxorubicin + methotrexate + 5-fluorouracil, CDV = cyclophosphamide + doxorubicin + vincristine, BDV = BCNU + DTIC + vincristine, PE = cisplatin + etoposide. Number of samples = patients has been presented.

Group	+++	++	+	+/-	-
Control	16	8	6	1	1
CDP	0	2	8	10	10
DMF	0	1	12	7	12
CDV	0	1	6	11	11
BDV	0	1	8	14	8
PE	1	0	17	8	5

The immunological reactions are seen in large extent in control animals only. In animals receiving cytotoxic therapy the immunological defence reactions are negligible. The whole problem of rejection is thus limited to animals which are necessarily not used in the evaluation of the assay. Further, there was no significant correlation between the extent of inflammation and tumor size change. It seems therefore that immunological reactions take place in the tumor pieces at least in lung cancer samples, but they have no clear influence on the evaluation. In gynecological cancers the immunological rejection seems to have markedly less , if any importance. Infiltration and inflammation reactions thus are dependent on the properties of each tumor.

The rejection can be avoided in control animals by immunosuppressive pretreatment like radiation, cytotoxic drugs or immunosuppressive drugs. Taking in account the minor importance of rejection in drug treated animals the benefit of pretreatment might be small. Perhaps a better solution could be addition of a second control group, properly immunosuppressed. Another possibility is to shorten the assay time from 6 to 4 days (Lévi et al, 1985). In this modification the evaluation has to be based on histology, not on size measurement.

4. Evaluation based on simple tumor size measurement by stereomicroscope is certainly rather rough estimate of drug effects. The major advantages of the method are simplicity, rapidity and that laboratory technicians can carry out the evaluation. The clinical evaluation is also based on tumor size measurement – the analogy to SRCA is exciting. The only published alternative to size measurement is histological evaluation. It is tedious, time consuming and requires a well trained pathologist. Unfortunately such pathologists are very seldom available. It is therefore presumed that routine SRCA cannot be based on histological evaluation. Other possibilities might be: vital staining and evaluation of unfixed samples, BrdUr given to the animals before final evaluation and subsequent flow cytometry as well as use of suitable radioactive precursors which penetrate into the actively growing tumor. None of these alternatives have been studied sufficiently. Conclusion: size measurement is the basic method. It should be compared to other methods. In problematic cases histological analysis is of great help. Active research is needed to improve the evaluation.

CLINICAL EXPERIENCES

Ovarian Cancer

The success rate of SRCA in ovarian cancer is very high, in our studies 123 out of 126 samples (98%). Also the histological analysis of the samples after the assay has shown that pieces contain a lot of living tumor cells and that inflammation reactions are not marked. Ovarian cancer therefore seems to be well evaluable. In retrospective studies with secondary laparotomy or CT controlled clinical response the concordance of SRCA result has been about 80% (table 2). It appears that all failed predictions except one are intermediate responses in SRCA and PD clinically. How—

ever, most patients in this group had only one or two
courses of treatment and the clinical efficacy of the therapy is not well evaluable. So we are not sure if we have
overestimated the response in SRCA slightly. Different combinations of cytotoxic drugs have been tested. Standard
chemotherapy in Finland (doxorubicin, cisplatin and cyclophosphamide) has been an effective combination but there
were several almost similar combinations. For the secondary
treatment at least the following combinations were promising: melphalan + cisplatin + hexamethylmelamine and cisplatin + etoposide + hexamethylmelamine. We have started a
prospective clinical trial with two treatment groups, one
receiving standard chemotherapy (doxorubicin, cisplatin,
cyclophosphamide) another SRCA directed chemotherapy. Disease free period and 5 year survival will be compared.

TABLE 2. Concordance of SRCA and clinical response in ovarian cancer. Sensitivity (S), intermediate sensitivity (I)
and resistance (R) in SRCA have been calculated according to
Mäenpää (1985). Number of patients in each group has been
indicated.

Clinical response	Evaluation in SRCA		
	S	I	R
CR	6	5	0
PR	3	5	1
NC	1	7	0
PD	0	10	4

In the prospective lung cancer study, success rate was
30/33 (91%). Chemotherapy to the patients was randomly
either cisplatin + etoposide or SRCA directed. In this study
the tumor pieces were studied by histology after the assay.
The results have been presented in table 3 in respect to
tumor cell amount. The results of histological analysis and
SRCA in respect to drug sensitivity were strikingly similar
in the evaluable samples. However, tumor size measurement
gives a much better quantitative result and it is seldom
possible to rank the drug efficacy by histological analysis.
Although it is too early to evaluate the concordance of SRCA
and clinical results, the first evaluations are promising.
SRCA never failed in samples where histological analysis
showed plenty of tumor cells.

TABLE 3. SRCA vs. histological evaluation in lung cancer samples. Share of tumor cells in the sample has been classified after the assay from +++ = very good sample, lot of tumor cells to - = no tumor cells. Not evaluable sample in histology contained dividing cartilaginous cells. (R) = all these samples were classified as resistant. SRCA evaluation: not evaluable = tumor size decreased in control samples, evaluable = tumor size increased but variations in results, well evaluable = clear tumor growth and small variation.

SRCA	Histology, share of tumor cells in the sample					
	+++	++	+	+/-	-	Not evaluable
Not evaluable	0	0	0	1	3	
Evaluable	2	1	0	3	3	
Well evaluable	2	3	5	4	3(R)	1

Mesothelioma study was a retrospective comparison of SRCA result and clinical response. Success rate was 28/30 (93%). Almost all samples have been extremely resistant to chemotherapy both in SRCA and clinically. The test predicted correctly the response in 10 out of the 12 evaluable patients. In the other patients responses were minor (NC) and also clinically difficult to interpret.

In melanoma samples a comparison was carried out between SRCA and flow cytometry of the original sample. Growth of the tumor in SRCA correlated with the fraction of S-phase cells. This was a very interesting finding and indicated that sample selection for SRCA had been successful and that the influence of inflammation on SRCA evaluation was of no importance.

In gastrointestinal cancer SRCA may greatly benefit the patients. Although clinical responses are not available, the response rate in SRCA is highly interesting: addition of doxorubicin, cisplatin, mitomycin C or carboquone to sequential methotrexate + 5-fluorouracil (+ leucovorin) increases the SRCA response rate from about 20% with conventional 5-fluorouracil + doxorubicin + mitomycin C -combination to more than 50%. Selection of the sample is of utmost importance in GI cancers due to the infection risk. The sample should not be in contact with the lumen of the gut.

SRCA seems not to be suited for chemotherapy testing in infected samples, in necrotic and stroma-rich samples, and in testing hormonal agents.

CONCLUSION

Predictive tests are important approach in improving the quality of cancer chemotherapy. SRCA is one of the most reliable tests. Success rate is high and predictive value even with the present modification acceptable. Further studies on technical improvements and controlled clinical trials are needed and are going on.

REFERENCES

Cunningham D, Jack A, McMurdo DFS, Soukop M McArdle CS, Carter DC, Kaye SB (1986). The 6 day subrenal capsule assay is of no value with primary surgical explants from gastric cancer. Br J Cancer 54:519-523.
Edelstein MB, Fiebig HH, Smink T, van Putten LM. Schuchhardt C (1983). Comparison between macroscopic and microscopic evaluation of tumour responsiveness using the subrenal capsule assay. Eur J Cancer Clin Oncol 19:995-1009.
Lévi F, Blum J-P, Lemaigre G, Mechkouri M, Roulon A, Mathé G (1985). A histological assessment of the four-day subrenal capsule assay (SRCA). Ann Chir Gynecol 74, Suppl 199:44-50.
Mäenpää J (1985). "The subrenal capsule assay in predicting responsiveness of gynecological cancers to drug therapy". Academic Dissertation, Turku University.

Prediction of Response to Cancer Therapy, pages 213-225
© 1988 Alan R. Liss, Inc.

THE CLINICAL USEFULNESS OF HUMAN XENOGRAFTS IN NUDE MICE

Tetsuro Kubota, Kyuya Ishibiki and Osahiko Abe

Department of Surgery, School of Medicine,
Keio University, Shinjuku-ku, Tokyo 160,
Japan

INTRODUCTION

Since the report of Povlsen and Rygaard (1971), many
papers have been published concerning experimental cancer
chemotherapy against human tumor xenografts serially
transplanted into nude mice. In these reports, it has
been elucidated that chemosensitivty of transferable
tumors is preserved from the original patients (Kubota et
al., 1978) and the chemosensitivity of each tumor is
constant throughout serial transplantations (Kubota et
al., 1983) as well as histolدgical features (Shimosato et
al., 1976), hormone dependency (Hirohashi et al., 1977)
and cell kinetics (Kubota et al., 1986). Although this
stable chemosensitivity of human tumor xenografts was
thought to be a suitable model for human cancer
chemotherapy, this model was difficult to apply clinically
to detect the chemosensitiivity of individual patients.
This was partly due to the reason that the mice are
expensive, it takes a lدt of time to establish a stable
strain that is adequate for chemotherapeutic experiments,
and overall take rates of primary transplantation are less
than 50% (Shimosato et al., 1976).

However, the human tumor xenograft - nude mouse
system is an excellent model to maintain a large amount of
tumor cells in vivo and supply them for experiments
constantly and repeatedly. If human tumor xenografts
represent the chemosensitive character of their original
organs and this chemosensitivity is not changed by serial
transplantations, this experimental model might be thought

to be suitable for use as a screening system to evaluate new antitumor agents. In this paper, we have tested chemosensitivity patterns of 21 human tumor xenografts to six antitumor agents to study whether this human tumor xenograft - nude mouse system might be adequate for screening new antitumor agents.

MATERIALS AND METHODS

Mice

BALB/c male and female nude mice originating from the Central Institute for Experimental Animals, Kawasaki, Japan, were purchased from CLEA Japan Inc., Tokyo, Japan. Male mice were used for the experiment except for breast carcinomas which were transplanted into female mice. Mice were kept under specific pathogen free conditions using laminar air flow racks in the experimental animal center of our institute, and were fed sterile food and water <u>ad libitum</u>. Six- to eight-week-old mice weighing 20-22 g were used for the experiment. Mice were weighed three times a week and their conditions were observed.

Tumors

Twenty one tumors used for the experiment are shown in Table 1 with their organs of origin and histological findings.

Tumors used were ten gastric, five breast, three colon and three lung small cell carcinomas. H-111 and SCK-29 were kindly provided from Dr. M. Fujita, Osaka University, and Dr. S. Takao, Kagoshima University, respectively. SC-2-JCK and SC-6-JCK were established at the Central Institute for Experimental Animals, Kawasaki and were provied by Dr. K. Maruo of that institute. MX-1 was established by Giovanella and was provided by Dr. K. Inoue, Cancer Chemotherapy Center, Tokyo. T-61 was provided from Dr. N. Brunner, Copenhagen University, Denmark. The other strains were established in the Pathology Division, the National Cancer Center Research Institute and in our department. All of these tumors were maintained in our institute by serial transplantation into nude mice. Because the growth of Br-10 in untreated

female mice was not sufficient for the chemotherapeutic
experiment and MCF-7 does not grow in untreated female
mice, 5 mg of 17ß-estradiol dipropionate and 250 mg of 17
-hydroxy progesterone caproate per kg were administered
once (Br-10) or three times (MCF-7) as reported previously
(Kubota et al., 1983).

Table 1. Tumors Used for the Experiments

organ	Tumor	Histology
stomach	St- 4	poorly differentiated adenocarcinoma
	St-10	well differentiated adenocarcinoma
	St-15	mucinous adenocarcinoma
	St-40	well differentiated adenocarcinoma
	H-111	well differentiated adenocarcinoma
	SCK-29	moderately differentiated adenocarcinoma
	SC-2-JCK	papillary or mucinous adenocarcinoma
	SC-6-JCK	moderately differentiated adenocarcinoma
	Exp-4	poorly differentiated adenocarcinoma
breast	MCF-7	common ductal carcinoma
	R- 27	common ductal carcinoma
	Br-10	common ductal carcinoma
	T- 61	common ductal carcinoma
	MX- 1	common ductal carcinoma
colon	Co- 3	well differentiated adenocarcinoma
	Co- 4	poorly differentiated adenocarcinoma
	Exp-42	mucinous adenocarcinoma
lung	Lu-24	small cell carcinoma
	Lu-130	small cell carcinoma
	Lu-134	small cell carcinoma

Drugs

Commercially available mitomycin C (MMC),
adriamycin (ADM), aclarubicin (ACR), 5-fluorouracil (5-
FU), cyclⅠphosphamide (CPA) and cisplatin (CDDP) were
used. MMC, ADM and 5-FU were purchased from Kyowa Hakko
Kogyo Co. Ltd., Tokyo. ACR, CPA and CDDP were purchased
from Yamanouchi Pharmaceutical Co. Ltd., Tokyo, Shionogi
and Co. Ltd., Osaka and Bristol Japan, Co. Ltd., Tokyo,
respectively. All of the drugs were dissolved in 0.2 ml
of 0.9% NaCl solution and were administered ip except ADM
which was given iv. Drugs were usually administered at a

schedule of q4dx3 except for CDDP which was given once. The treatment was started when the estimated tumor weight reached 100-300 mg as described later.

The doses of drugs, schedule and route of administration are summarized in Table 2. The doses were the maximum tolerated ones of each agent in nude mice, as determined in our institute.

Table 2. Drugs Used for the Experiment

Drug	Dose	Schedule	Route
mitomycin C (MMC)	3 mg/kg	q4dx3	ip
adriamycin (ADM)	4 mg/kg	q4dx3	iv
aclarubicin (ACR)	10 mg/kg	q4dx3	ip
cyclophosphamide (CPA)	80 mg/kg	q4dx3	ip
5-fluorouracil (5-FU)	50 mg/kg	q4dx3	ip
cisplatin (CDDP)	9 mg/kg	qdx1	ip

Tumor Inoculations Measurement of Tumor Size and Evaluation of Drug Activity

Two tissue fragments of approximately 3x3x3 mm in size were inoculated into the subcutaneous tissue of the dorsum of ether anesthetized nude mice by mean of trocar needle. Tumors were measured (length and width) with sliding calipers three times weekly by the same observer.

According to the method of Geran et al. (1972), the tumor weight in mg was calculated from the linear measurements using the formula: tumor weight (mg) = length (mm) x (width(mm))^2/2.

When tumor reached 100-300 mg, tumor bearing mice were randomized into test groups consisting of four to six mice each. The relative mean tumor weight (RW) was calculated as RW = Wi/Wo, where Wi was the mean tumor weight at any given time and Wo is the mean tumor weight at the initial treatment. The antitumor effect of the drugs were evaluated by the lowest T/C ratio (%) during the experiment, where T was the relative mean tumor weight of the treated group and C the relative mean tumor weight of the control group at any given time. The antitumor activity was evaluated as positive when the lowest T/C was equal or less than 42%, which was calculated from $(0.75)^3$ meaning a 25% reduction of each diameter.

Statistical Analysis

The efficiency rate of drug in human tumor xenograft - nude mouse system was compared with the clinically reported efficiency rate of the same drug (Carter and Friedman, 1974, Comis and Carter, 1974 and Carter, 1976). The coefficient of correlation was calculated between the efficiency rates in nude mouse system and that in clinical reports, and was statistically examined by t-test.

RESULTS

The antitumor activities of the drugs against human gastric carcinoma xenografts are shown in Table 3.

TABLE 3.   Antitumor Activity of Drugs against Human Gastric Carcinoma Xenografts

Tumor	MMC	ADM	ACR	CPA	5-FU	CDDP	Response rate
St -4	65.0	48.3	46.3	45.6	87.6	91.7	0%
St-10	13.0£	28.4£	35.5£	72.7	ND	41.0£	80%
St-15	22.7£	66.2	56.7	51.5	61.4	27.2£	33.3%
St-40	7.3£	64.9	52.5	64.9	98.1	23.6£	33.3%
H-111	45.5	54.4	44.0	51.0	31.3£	67.8	16.7%
KS- 1	12.1£	24.3£	35.1£	73.7	ND	ND	75%
SCK-29	77.2	63.9	ND	27.5£	ND	ND	33.3%
SC-2-JCK	18.0£	69.4	ND	44.8	56.2	29.4£	40%
SC-6-JCK	5.2£	78.4	ND	72.0	39.0£	17.0£	60%
Exp-4	37.0£	63.5	ND	47.0	50.3	19.1£	40%
Efficacy rate (%)	70	20	33.3	10	28.6	75	39.2%

£.T/C less than 42%
Data were shown as the lowest T/C ratio during the experiment.
ND: not done

In six antitumor drugs tested, CDDP showed a most excellent antitumor activity with an efficiency rate of 75%, followed by MMC of which efficiency rate was 70%.

CPA was ineffective against 9 of 10 gastric carcinoma xenografts. The efficiency rates of ADM, ACR and 5-FU ranged from 20 to 33.3%. From the viewpoint of sensitivity pattern of xenografts, no drugs were effective on St-4, and H-111 was sensitive only to 5-FU. On the other hand, St-10, KS-1 and SC-6-JCK were found to be sensitive to most of tested drugs, suggesting a variety of sensitivity of human gastric carcinoma xenografts.

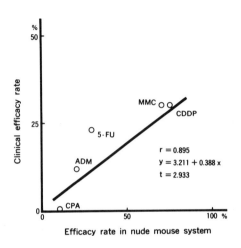

Figure 1. Efficiency Rate of Drugs against Gastric Carcinomas in Nude Mouse and Human

Figure 1 shows the correlation between the efficiency rate of antitumor drugs in human tumor xenograft - nude mouse system and that in clinical reports (Comis and Carter, 1974, and Japanese early phase II trial of CDDP on gastric carcinoma). The clinical efficiency rates of CDDP and MMC which were effective against human gastric carcinoma xenografts, are reported to be 30% in clinical reports, whereas CPA which was ineffective on 9 of 10 xenografts, is reported to have no value on patients with gastric carcinoma. The efficiency rates of ADM and 5-FU were observed to be intermediate value between these three drugs. The coefficient of correlation between the efficiency rates in nude mouse system and clinical reports were 0.895 with a statistical significance. Antitumor spectra of tested drugs against human breast carcinoma xenografts were shown in Table 4.

TABLE 4. Antitumor Activity of the Drugs against Human Breast Carcinoma Xenografts

Tumor	MMC	ADM	ACR	CPA	5-FU	CDDP	Response rate
MCF-7	23.4£	64.5	65.7	36.3£	63.5	ND	40%
R- 27	11.7£	70.5	ND	36.3£	ND	ND	66.7%
Br-10	21.0£	90.0	42.8	30.9£	89.3	ND	40%
T- 61	44.1	52.0	ND	21.4£	ND	ND	33.3%
MX- 1	7.9£	39.8£	19.7£	0.8£	52.4	3.4£	83.3%
Eff. rate	80%	20%	33.3%	100%	0%	1/1	54.5%

£T/C less than 42%
Data were shown as the lowest T/C ratio during the experiment.
ND: not done

In breast carcinoma xenografts, CPA and MMC showed high antitumor activity with efficiency rates of 5/5 and 4/5, respectively. It was obvious that CPA which was ineffective on 9 of 10 gastric carcinoma xenografts were effective against all of breast carcinoma xenografts tested. Whereas ADM was found to effective on 20% of breast carcinoma xenografts, no tumors were sensitive to 5-FU. From the viewpoint of sensitivity pattern of each xenograft, hormone independent MX-1 was highly sensitive to all of drugs tested except 5-FU, and the complete regressions of the treated tumors were observed by CPA and CDDP.

Antitumor activity of drugs against three colon carcinoma xenografts were shown in Table 5.

CPA which was ineffective on gastric carcinoma xenografts, was also ineffective on colon carcinomas, while all of breast carcinomas were sensitive to this drug. Co-4 established from a cultured cell line C-1 was sensitive to 3 of 5 drugs including 5-FU which was ineffective on MX-1. Whereas all over efficiency rate on colon carcinomas was 35.3%, this rate was decreased until 18.2% when Co-4 was excluded.

TABLE 5. Antitumor Activity of Drugs against Human Colдn Carcinoma Xenografts

Tumor	MMC	ADM	ACR	CPA	5-FU	CDDP	Response rate
Co- 3	71.9	55.4	37.4£	92.0	44.8	ND	20%
Co- 4	13.8£	52.1	26.4£	81.0	13.4£	15.8£	66.7%
Exp-42	41.9£	44.4	79.7	74.9	68.0	73.4	16.7%
Eff. rate (%)	66.7	0	66.7	0	33.3	50	35.3%

£T/C less than 42%
Data were shown as the lдwest T/C ratio during the experiment.
ND: not done

The efficiency rates of drugs in human tumor - nude mouse system and clinical reports were compared in Table 6.

TABLE 6. Efficacy Rate of Drugs against Human Tumor Xenografts and Clinical Tumors

Tumor		MMC	ADM	CPA	5-FU	CDDP	r
stomach	mouse	70	20	10	28.5	75	0.895
	human	30	12	0	23	30	
breast	mouse	80	20	100	0	ND	0.670
	human	38	35	34	26	ND	
colдn	mouse	66.7	0	0	33.3	ND	-0.215
	human	16	12	27	21	ND	

Data were shown as efficiency rate in %.

Although good correlation was observed in gastric carcinoma, the correlation in breast carcinoma is not enough and no correlation was present in colдn carcinomas.
Table 7 shows the antitumor activity of agents against lung small cell carcinoma xenografts. While lung small cell carcinoma is known to be one of the most sensitive carcinomas to antitumor agents, the overall response rate of small cell carcinoma xenografts was only 40% which was not so different from the response rates of digestive and breast carcinoma xenografts. CDDP which is one of the key drugs on small cell carcinomas is under-

estimated in nude mouse system and 5-FU which is less effective on this cancer showed a remarkable antitumor effect against Lu-134. These data suggested that lung small cell carcinoma xenografts can not represent the characteristics of chemosensitivity of small cell carcinomas in human beings.

TABLE 7. Antitumor Activity of Drugs against Lung Small Cell Carcinomas

Tumor	MMC	ADM	CPA	5-FU	CDDP	Response rate
Lu- 24	20.4£	33.3£	8.3£	68.0	65.6	60%
Lu-130	6.4£	66.1	76.1	90.6	86.8	20%
Lu-134	4.4£	63.0	61.5	1.4£	42.6	40%
Eff. rate (%)	100	33.3	33.3	33.3	0	40%

£T/C less than 42%
Data were shown as the lowest T/C ratio during the experiment.

DISCUSSION

If chemosensitivity of the transferable strain in nude mice represents the characteristics seen in the organs of origin, it was assumed that this human tumor xenograft - nude mouse system was suitable as a screening model for new antitumor agents. This paper deals with the chemosensitivity of each strain, and their chemosensitivity pattern was compared with that of clinically reported cases.

Although some variety of chemosensitivity pattern in the carcinomas originated from the same organ was obtained, the overall sensitivity patterns of breast carcinoma and digestive carcinoma were different to each other, where CPA was effective on 5 of 5 breast carcinomas, while only 1 of 13 digestive carcinomas was sensitive to CPA.

Actually, the correlation of chemosensitivity between human xenografts and clinical patients was positive in gastric and breast carcinomas, where more effective drugs on human xenografts are reported to be effective on patients with gastric and breast carcinomas. However, the correlation of chemosensitivity between nude mouse system and clinical report was not excellent in coll|n and lung small cell carcinomas. In colon carcinoma xenografts, only Co-4 was sensitive to most of drugs tested and the remaining two strains were insensitive to the drugs. Co-4 is originated from a cultured cell line C-1 which was established from a metastatic lesion of colon carcinoma. As this strain was cultured in vitro for several years, any mutation might occur concerning with its chemosensitivity. It is well known that the chemosensitivity of colon carcinomas are relatively low, and less susceptibility of the remaining two strains could represent the chemosensitive character of colon carcinomas in human beings. As for small cell carcinomas, we have already reported that the cell kinetics of small cell carcinoma xenografts in nude mouse is different from that of digestive carcinomas (Kubota et al, 1985). Furthermore, the take rate of this carcinoma is reported to be low (Shimosato et al., 1976), in spite of rapid growth rate of this tumor in human beings. These findings might suggest any incomplete adaptation of small cell carcinomas to nude mouse and this differnt mode of growth rate of small cell carcinoma in nude mouse might be one of the reasons for different chemosensitivity of this tumor in nude mouse.

From these considerations, we have concluded that the gastric and breast carcinoma xenografts would be a promising model to screen a novel antitumor agents before clinical phase II study. Figure 2 shows the schema to use the human tumor xenograft - nude mouse system as a preclinical screening system for a newly developed antitumor agent. When a novel drug was certified its antitumor activity by rodent tumor panels or cultured human tumor cells in vitro, the agent would be tested by Co-4 and MX-1. As, in our experiments, no drugs were effective against any other human tumor xenografts when the drug was ineffective on MX-1 or Co-4, these two strains were thought to be adequate as a primary screening target. After this primary screening, the new agent could enter the secondary panel of gastric or breast carcinomas where we can orient the disease on which the clinical phase II study should be performed. By orienting the disease through this procedure, it will be possible to avoid a useless and harmful phase II study in the clinics.

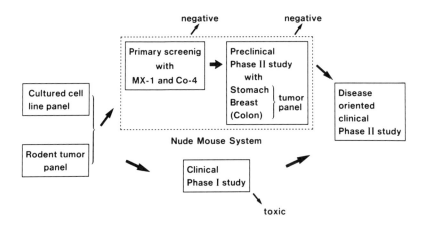

Figure 2. Human Xenografts as Preclinical Phase II

This secondary screening of human xenografts could be said as a "preclinical phase II study". However, it should be emphasized that this system is not a "preclinical phase I study", because nude mouse with immune deficiency is not an appropriate model to evaluate and predict the toxicity of drugs in human patient. Preclinical animal toxicity test or phase I test using patients with advanced carcinomas should be investigated in parallel with this preclinical phase II study. Furthermore, pharmacokinetic data from patients in phase I study should be used to determine the dose which will be tested in human tumor xenografts – nude mouse system to increase the correlation of efficiency rates between nude mouse system and clinical results, as reported elsewhere (Inaba et al., 1984).

In our institue, some compounds are under investigation of this preclinical and clinical phase II study. They are carboplatin and quinocarmycin against gastric carcinomas and KM2210, a conjugate of estradiol and chlorambucil (Kubota et al., 1986) against breast carcinomas. Actually, KM2210 which was evaluated as positive against 6 of 13 human xenografts including complete regression of MX-1, showed an efficiency rate of 33.3% against clinical breast carcinomas in Phae II study (Abe et al., 1986).

ACKNOWLEDGEMENT

This work was supported in part by Grants-in-Aids from the Ministry of Education, Science and Culture and Ministry of Health and Welfare, Japan. The authors would like to thank doctors of the Mickey Mouse Club of our department who cooperated in these experiments.

REFERENCES

Abe O, Izuo M, Watanabe H, Enomoto K, Ohsawa N, Kuno K (1986). Early phase II study of bestrabucil on advanced recurrent breast cancer. Oncoldgia 18:158-166. (in Japanese)

Carter SK, Friedman M (1974). Integration of chemotherapy into combined modality treatment of solid tumors. II. large bowel carcinoma. Cancer Treat Reviews 1:111-129.

Carter SK (1976). Cancer treatment today and its impact on drug develdpment, with special emphasis on the phase II clinical trial. J Natl Cancer Inst 57:235-244.

Comis RL, Carter SK (1974). Integration of chemotherapy into combined modality treatment of solid tumors. III. gastric cancer. Cancer Treat Reviews 1:221-238.

Geran RI, Greenberg NH, Macdonald MM, Schumacher AM, Abbott BJ (1972). Protocols for screening chemical agents and natural products against animal tumors and other biolΙΙgical systems (third edition). Cancer Chemother Rep 3:51-61.

Hirohashi S, Shimosato Y, Kameya T, Nagai K, Tsunematsu R (1977). Hormone dependency of a serially transplantable human breast cancer (Br-10) in nude mice. Cancer Res 37:3184-3189.

Inaba M, Tashiro T, Kobayashi T, Fujimoto S, Sakurai Y, Maruo K, Saito M, Ueyama Y, Nomura T (1984). Responsiveness of human tumor xenografts to chemotherapy with special reference to clinical dose. In Sordat B (ed): "Immune-Deficient Animals", Basel: Karger, pp 421-424.

Kubota T, Shimosato Y, Nagai K (1978). Experimental chemotherapy of carcinoma of the human stomach and colön serially transplanted into nude mice. Gann 69:299-309.

Kubota T, Hanatani Y, Tsuyuki K, Nakada M, Ishibiki K, Abe O, Kamataki T, Kato R (1983). Antitumor effect and metabolic activation of cyclöphosphamide and 4-OOH-cyclophosphamide in the human breast carcinoma (MX-1) - nude mouse system. Gann 74:437-444.

Kubota T, Kubouchi K, Koh J, Enomoto K, Ishibiki K, Abe O (1983). Human breast carcinoma (MCF-7) serially transplanted into nude mice. Jpn J Surg 13:381-384.

Kubota T, Inada T, Nakada M, Tsuyuki K, Ishibiki K, Abe O (1985). Cell kinetics of human lung small cell carcinomas transplanted into nude mice. Jpn J Cancer Chemother 12:1775-1781. (in Japanese)

Kubota T, Nakada M, Tsuyuki K, Inada T, Asanuma F, Ishibiki K, Abe O (1986). Cell kinetics and chemosensitivity of human carcinomas serially transplanted into nude mice. Jpn J Cancer Res (Gann) 77:502-507.

Kubota T, Kawamura E, Suzuki T, Yamada T, Toyoda H, Miyagawa T, Kurokawa T (1986). Jpn J Clin Oncol 16:357-364.

Povlsen CO, Rygaard J (1971). Heterotransplantation of a human adenocarcinoma of the colön and rectum to the mouse mutant nude, A study of nine consequtive transplantations. Acta pathol Microbiol Scand A 79:159-169.

Shimosato Y, Kameya T, Nagai K, Hirohashi S, Koide T, Hayashi H, Nomura T (1976). Transplantation of human tumors in nude mice. J Natl Cancer Inst 56:1251-1260.

Prediction of Response to Cancer Therapy, pages 227–235
© 1988 Alan R. Liss, Inc.

THE USE OF CLINICAL DATA TO PREDICT RESPONSE TO THERAPY

Emil J Freireich

Adult Leukemia Research Program, The University of
Texas System Cancer Center, M.D. Anderson Hospital
and Tumor Institute, Houston, Texas 77030

The most powerful tool for predicting natural
history and response to therapy for malignant disease is
the analysis of clinical data already known to affect
prognosis. It is generally appreciated among physicians,
that the most important technique for assessing prognosis
and assigning treatment is accurate diagnosis. It is
hardly surprising to recognize that patients who have
estrogen receptors on their tumor cells are much more
likely to respond if their cancer is classified as
originating from the female breast as opposed to those
arising from cancer of the colon or melanoma. Moreover,
it has long been realized that the stage of the disease,
that is the degree of spread outside of the site of
origin is always highly significant in prognosis and
response to treatment. The prototypic example is those
tumors which arise in a site and are confined in that
site are frequently referred to as stage I. Such tumors
are regularly cured with locally ablative treatment such
as surgery or radiation. In contrast, tumors which are
widely metastatic but have the same histopathology and
organ of origin, etc., have the other extreme, virtually
no response to such treatment and a poor prognosis. Thus
it is generally appreciated that for every diagnosis,
there is in addition a diagnosis-specific staging system
which assists in predicting the natural history of the
untreated disease and this is the most important factor
in predicting response to treatment.

WHAT CLINICAL VARIABLES ARE IMPORTANT FOR PREDICTING RESPONSE?

In addition to diagnosis and stage, at the time of diagnosis of malignancy, the clinician collects an enormous wealth of additional objective and subjective information about the patient. In our own experience when we analyzed the number of observations that were made in a single patient with the diagnosis of adult acute leukemia, we found that this number was in excess of 300. Of these single variables, if correlations of each taken one at a time are made with prognosis, we found that there were over 50 that were highly correlated with prognosis and with response to treatment. The medical literature is full of such analyses of variables which predict for outcome and investigators have for years arbitrarily or intuitively selected those variables which they choose to be used in predicting response to treatment. The breast cancer example serves very well in this regard since we know that in addition to diagnosis and stage, there is menopausal status, duration from primary to recurrent disease, nuclear grade, invasion of lymphatics, degree of fibrosis, etc. The difficulty with predicting response from clinical variables is not because of a deficiency of knowledge, but because of an excess of knowledge and the lack of a relatively simple and systematic way to organize such knowledge.

MULTIVARIATE STATISTICAL METHODS FOR ANALYZING CLINICAL VARIABLES

There are a number of statistical techniques which allow the simplification of complex data to render it more manageable and interpretable. One useful technique is the use of stepwise forward regression analysis to accomplish an ordering of those variables which contribute the most information to statements about prognosis and perhaps more important to create the ordering in such a way that each variable adds knowledge independent of the preceding one chosen to be important (Estey, 1984). Although the technique has been expounded much more lucidly by much better informed authors, nonetheless the general strategy is to examine the degree of correlation between all single variables and whatever is being chosen for prognosis, be it survival, response to treatment, etc. Then one objectively ranks all

individual variables and decides that the one that has
the best quantitative correlation with the existing data
set will be chosen as the single most important variable.
It is important to emphasize that such choices are
arbitrary. A good analogy is a track and field event
where a large number of individuals run in a given day in
a given race, the one who finishes first is called the
winner although he is not necessarily going to win every
race when the same individuals run. Nonetheless one can
arbitrarily decide that that person is the best and
future competitions to establish a better runner will
require someone superior to that individual.

Once a variable is chosen, the next question to be
investigated is which of all the remaining variables, if
added as a single variable to the one chosen as the best,
would provide the greatest increase in predictive power
or stated another way, would account for a greater part
of the observed variability in outcome. Again, all the
remaining variables are ordered by that criteria and the
one that wins is chosen as second and then we proceed to
find a third by investigating the question, which of the
remaining add to the first two. It is not necessary to
order all the variables since there is always strong
correlation of variables with each other. What generally
happens is that as you proceed in a stepwise fashion to
add subsequent variables, you reach a point when the next
variable chosen that contributes most to the ones already
chosen, does not significantly improve the ability to
predict outcome. At that point the stepwise forward
regression analysis can stop. In our experience,
depending on the size of the data base, only a very
limited number of variables will emerge, somewhere
between three and six, after which additional information
is not useful. The result is an identification in a
quantitative way of those variables which predict for
outcome. Perhaps the most important property of such
procedures is that it can be totally objective, that is
you can allow the computer to create a table ordering
those variables most useful for predicting outcome
(Estey, 1987).

MODELS FOR PREDICTING RESPONSE

Once the stepwise forward logistic regression
analysis is completed, it is new possible to generate a

model based on the identified variables which predict in
a quantitative way the probability of patients' response.
From the analysis one can create a logistic regression
equation which provides factors to assign to the variable
for each individual patient. Thus for example, we have
generated a model which uses six factors which predicts
for response for any given individual. Then the
objective quantitative measure of those six variables,
can be entered into the equation derived from the large
data base, and compute an exact prediction for that
individual. This can take the form of probability of
response to a given treatment or it could be a continuous
variable such as duration of survival or response by
using a slightly different procedure (Freireich, 1983).

TESTING OF MODELS

From any given data set where outcomes are known,
for example, response to treatment, after a logistic
regression model is created the first test of the
usefulness of such a model would be to apply the model
generated from analysis of the variables within the
entire group of patients to the data base from which it
was derived. That is, for each patient in the data base,
a probability of response can be computed with the model
and then one can examine with a variety of statistical
techniques how well the model functions when applied to
the individual patients from whom the model was derived.
Since the theoretical basis for the modeling procedures
is quite good, this test is almost regularly an easy
test to pass, that is most logistic regression models
perform very well when applied to the data base from
which it was derived (Freireich, 1974).

The next step is to test the model in prospect.
This is accomplished by assigning exact probabilities to
each patient before treatment is applied and then to
analyze the observed outcomes to be compared to the
predicted ones. If the model performs well in the
prospective test, this provides strong evidence that such
modeling would be useful for future application. Another
important feature of the prospectively validated model is
that the investigator now has more assurance that such
modeling can be useful for evaluating a candidate new
treatment. It is important to emphasize that each
analysis has to be specific for the treatment for which

predictions have been made and when a new treatment is to
be evaluated, a hypothesis to be evaluated in prospect
would be, is the candidate new treatment equal to or
better than the outcome for a given set of patients would
have been with a conventional treatment. Then it is
possible to create ratios between observed outcomes and
expected outcomes for a group of patients treated
consecutively on a given treatment. This has proven to
be a powerful technique for conducting phase II type
studies. It is particularly useful where the expectation
for benefit from conventional treatment is low
(Freireich, 1973).

ASSIGNING TREATMENT BASED ON PREDICTED PROBABILITY OF
RESPONSE

In the circumstance where existing treatment is
highly effective, but like any treatment, not perfect,
the modeling procedures can also be extremely useful. For
instance, it is possible to arbitrarily select favorable
response probabilities where new treatment would have
little likelihood of improving response and investigating
new treatments only in patient groups that have lower
probabilities of response. Thus it is possible to assign
patients to treatments based on predicted outcome from
known treatments. In this way, the patients who have the
most favorable responses are protected from the potential
hazards of an innovative treatment while at the same
time, patients with low probabilities of response to
existing treatment have the benefit of potentially better
treatment at the same time they are exposed to the
increased risk from unknown effects of the new treatment.
This experimental plan has proven to be extremely useful
and highly efficient in phase III studies where
treatments known to be effective in advanced stages are
offered to patients with earlier stages of disease
(Gehan, 1981).

ADDITION OF NEW INFORMATION

When a new procedure or a new regimen becomes
available, an important question is, does the new
information significantly improve our ability to predict
response. This new information could be some in vitro
tests, sensitivity of the tumor to a drug, or it might be
a new measurement that relates to the tumor, such as the

cytogenetics in the case of acute leukemia (Gehan, 1980). This question again can be addressed with these statistical methods. The best known model for predicting response to available therapy can be augmented by including the new fact in a stepwise forward regression analysis and see if it wins in any of the races, that is whether it comes in a position where it adds substantially to existing knowledge better than the already identified variables. If it does appear, this is strong evidence that this variable is important in improving the quality of the predictions and it is an important addition to the known clinical variables. On the other hand, if it does not enter as important, it is still possible to test the impact of a new test by entering it in the model as the first variable and seeing whether the other known clinical variables are affected. For a new test which adds nothing substantial by starting with that as your first test, the other clinical variables would appear in roughly the order and degree of association that they did before and it would be obvious that the test added little or nothing. At the other extreme, if the test was quite important, it would be obvious that the variables which added to the knowledge you already had from that test would be different and in different order. A striking example of the latter is with the description of unique banded cytogenetic aneuploidies in acute myeloblastic leukemia (Holmes, 1985). When we started with the knowledge of cytogenetic aneuploidy, the variables which added to that were uniquely different and the quality of the prediction was greatly improved. It was obvious from this study that the banded cytogenetics was an extremely important variable in predicting response to a given treatment and in predicting overall outcome for the patients. Subsequently unique clinical and biological features were found to be associated with these cytogenetic patterns (Keating, 1987).

Thus the models useful for predicting response can be continuously upgraded, and improved in quality with the discovery of new testing procedures, and the model allows the investigator to investigate whether a new test adds significantly to the existing ability to predict response.

TREATMENT EFFECTS

In addition to predicting response and survival based on clinical characteristics present at the time of diagnosis, modeling procedures can be useful in subsequent phases of disease. For example, in the case of acute myelogenous leukemia, the prognosis for patients who responded to induction, that is, patients who are now in complete hematological remission, the prediction of who will remain in remission for the longest time or alternatively, which are cured, requires a different approach. Therefore if an analysis is confined to those patients who achieved complete remission, quite different variables will appear than were present in the original model predicting for probability of response (Keating, 1987). There are a number of reasons for that which are evident, but the most obvious one is that the patient samples are quite different. All the poor prognosis patients have failed to achieve remission and are removed from the denominator and more important, there are treatment effects which enter into the modeling. In the case of acute leukemia, it was found that the speed of induction of complete remission, that is the time from onset of treatment to documenting complete disappearance of disease was a significant variable for predicting the quality of response or the duration of response. Undoubtedly this is due to the specific interaction of the treatment and the tumor. Knowledge which was not present at the time the patient's treatment was initiated.

In a similar vein, we had reported that for patients who are treated with a salvage or a second order treatment with acute leukemia, the variable which is most predictive for both response and survival is the duration of the first treatment, that is the quality of response to the first treatment is the best predictor for quality of response to subsequent treatments (Keating, 1980). Information in the salvage situation is added which could not be known until the patients were systematically exposed to a specific treatment. It must be remembered that each of these statements are treatment-specific, that is it depends on the treatment regimen being used. An analogy might be the circumstance for the treatment of localized breast cancer. The variables which predict for a successful conversion of a patient with localized

disease to a patient free of disease obviously relate to
the impact of surgery on the host. In contrast, the
variables which predict for the likelihood that a patient
then free of disease will have recurrent disease is
dominantly influenced by extent of disease at the time of
surgery, for instance, node involvement, estrogen
receptor status, etc (Smith, 1982).

Thus modeling based on clinical variables can be
useful at all stages of disease and they can be useful
for assigning treatment and for assessing outcome based
on predicted expectations compared to observed outcomes.

SUMMARY

Clinical data are useful for predicting response to
therapy and prognosis of patients with malignant disease.
Multivariate statistical methods have proven to be useful
for objectively evaluating those variables which are most
useful for predicting outcome. Once variables have been
identified, models can be created which predict for
individuals the expectations for response and survival
and such models with known clinical variables are useful
for evaluating the contribution of newly developed
information such as in vitro testing or a new laboratory
test in terms of its contribution to the ability to
predict response. The models are then useful for
evaluation of treatment effects by comparing observed
effects of new treatments to expectations for each
patient.

REFERENCES

Estey EH, Keating MJ, Smith TL, McCredie KB, Legha SS,
    Walters RS, Bodey GP, Freireich EJ (1984). Prediction
    of complete remission in patients with refractory acute
    leukemia treated with AMSA. J Clin Onc 2:102-106.
Estey E, Plunkett W, Dixon D, Keating M, McCredie K,
    Freireich EJ (1987). Variables predicting response to
    high dose cytosine arabinoside therapy in patients with
    refractory acute leukemia. Leukemia 1(8):580-583.
Freireich EJ (1983). Methods for evaluating response to
    treatment in adult acute leukemia. Blood Cells 9:5-20.

Freireich EJ, Gehan EA, Bodey GP, Hersh EM, Hart JS,
Gutterman JU, McCredie KB (1974). New prognostic
factors affecting response and survival in adult acute
leukemia. Transactions of the Association of the
American Physicians 87:298-305.
Freireich EJ, Gehan EA, Speer JF, Heilbrun L, Smith T,
Bodey GP, McCredie KB, Rodriguez V, Hart JS, Burgess
MA (1973). The usefulness of multiple pretreatment
patient characteristic for prediction of response and
survival in patients with adult acute leukemia.
Advances in the Biosciences 14:131-144.
Gehan EA, Freireich EJ (1981). Cancer Clinical Trials.
A rational basis for use of historical controls. Sem
in Onc 8(4):430-436.
Gehan EA, Smith TL, Buzdar AU, Keating MJ, Freireich EJ
(1980). Knowledge acquisition from historical data:
Application to breast cancer patients. Bull. Cancer
(Paris) 67:437-445.
Holmes R, Keating MJ, Cork A, Broach Y, Trujillo JM,
Dalton WT, McCredie KB, Freireich EJ (1985). A unique
pattern of central nervous system leukemia in acute
myelomonocytic leukemia associated with inv(16)
(p13q22). Blood 65(5):1071-1078.
Keating MJ, Cork A, Broach Y, Smith T, Walters RS,
McCredie KB, Trujillo J, Freireich EJ (1987). Toward a
clinically relevant cytogenetic classification of acute
myelogenous leukemia. Leukemia Res 11(2):119-133.
Keating MJ, Gehan EA, Smith TL, Estey EH, Walters RS,
Kantarjian HM, McCredie KB, Freireich EJ (1987). A
strategy for evaluation of new treatments in untreated
patients: Application to a clinical trial of AMSA for
acute leukemia. J Clin Onc 5:710-721.
Keating MJ, Smith TL, Gehan EA, McCredie KB, Bodey GP,
Spitzer G, Hersh E, Gutterman JU, Freireich EJ (1980).
Factors related to length of complete remission in
adult acute leukemia. Cancer 45:2017-2029.
Smith TL, Gehan EA, Keating MJ, Freireich EJ (1982).
Prediction of remission in adult acute leukemia.
Cancer 50:466-472.

Prediction of Response to Cancer Therapy, pages 237-254
© 1988 Alan R. Liss, Inc.

BIOCHEMICAL AND CYTOKINETIC CHARACTERIZATION OF
LEUKEMIC CELLS: PREDICTION OF TREATMENT RESULTS
AND EARLY DIAGNOSIS OF RELAPSE.

Wolfgang Wilmanns, Hansjörg Sauer,
Renate Pelka-Fleischer,Liane Twardzik,
Ursula Vehling-Kaiser.
Medical Clinic III, Ludwig-Maximilians-
Universität Munich and Institute of
Clinical Hematology GSF Munich,
West-Germany.

INTRODUCTION

In the treatment of acute leukemia with cytotoxic agents and corticosteroids not always the
desired therapeutic effect is achieved. In addition side effects on normal proliferating cells
may cause severe complications. Therefore efforts
to characterize acute leukemias for predicting
prognosis and response to treatment are of high
importance. Significant differences in prognosis
were found with clinical staging and laboratory
tests (1,3,5,24,28). Quantitative cytological
measurements of leukemic blasts and their biochemical and cytogenetic characterization (2,3,11,
13,20,27,30,33,34) and cytokinetic data of the
distribution of leukemic blast cells to different
phases in the cell-division-cycle (6,9,18,19,21)
showed some correlation with response to treatment
and different prognosis.

Stem-cell colony assays alone or together with
in vitro cytostatic drug sensitivity testing also
have been used for predicting the outcome of therapy (11,14,15,16,22). But these assays are time
consuming and not always reproducable.

We have investigated the DNA-synthesis in
leukemic cells under the action of different agents
in vitro and in vivo (31,32,33) and have correlated
the results with cytokinetic data. We have found

that in vitro investigations have high probability
of errors. This is understandable as by these in
vitro tests metabolic and regulative events, which
might be important for the action of cytotoxic
drugs in vivo, are not detected. In this respect
our results are not in accordance with other publications showing a correlation between in vitro
chemosensitivity to specific drugs and the quality
of response to treatment (7,12,23,29). At a time
when single drugs with cytotoxic action were
applied to leukemic patients the evaluation of the
sensitivity of leukemic cells could be highly improved if in vitro tests were completed by investigations in vivo within short time inverVals after
single injection of specific acting drugs (31,32,
33). Thus, concerning the reduction of leukemic
blast-cells, in each treated patient intensity
and duration of therapeutic effects could be evaluated within three days. It has to be stated in
this connection that the judgement of sensitivity
of the leukemic cell population to be treated is
not identical with the prognosis of remission.
A remission is not only dependent on the destruction of the leukemic cells but also on the regene-
ration of the hematopoesis from normal stem cells.

With the development of new therapeutic
strategies by applying intensive polychemotherapy
together with supportive care nearly all treated
patients come into an aplastic phase, and the remission rate is increased dramatically.

The aim of investigations, reported in this
presentation, was to look for markers suitable in
following the course of leukemic patients under
and after polychemotherapy, especially for early
detection of relapse. Another question was, as to
whether or not there is a possibility to predict
the treatment's outcome from the DNA metabolic activities at primary diagnosis and from changes
in these parameters during the very early phase of
treatment. To characterize the DNA metabolic activity in comparison to cell cycle parameters in normal and leukemic bone marrow specimens we determined quantitatively the incorporation of Thymidine
(dTR) and Deoxyuridine (dUR) into the DNA of intact

cells and the activity of Thymidine Kinase (TK) in
the cytosol using biochemical methods as well as
the %S-phase-cells in specifically DNA-stained
cells by a cytofluorometric method.

The biochemical pathways of DNA-synthesis
are shown in Figure 1.

NUCLEOSIDE-INCORPORATION

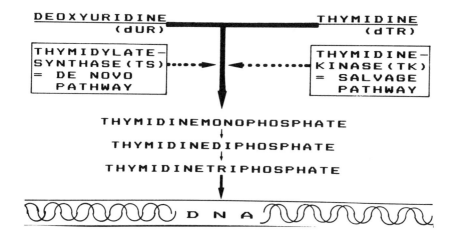

Figure 1. DNA-synthesis: selected pathways.

The incorporation-rates of the nucleosides
deoxyuridine (dUR) and deoxythymidine (dTR) represent two different metabolic pathways. In the de
novo pathway thymidinemonophosphate (dTMP) is synthesized in the folic-acid-dependent step of thymi-
dylate synthase (TS). In this reaction thymidine
kinase (TK) activity is not needed. The salvage
pathway uses preformed dTR, which is phosphorylated in the TK reaction. In proliferating cells
the identical reduplication of DNA occurs during
the DNA-synthesis phase (S-phase) of the cell
cycle.

MATERIAL AND METHODS

Bone marrow specimens

Bone marrow was taken mostly from the iliac crest and from the sternum when iliac crest puncture was not possible. 1 ml of bone marrow was aspirated and mixed with 0,2 ml of phosphate buffered saline (0,9% NACl in 0,0007 M K-phosphate buffer pH 7,4; w/v) containing 1% Mg-EDTA (w/v) and 2% D-glucose (w/v).

395 marrow specimens were assayed: 26 from normal controls, 103 from patients with acute leukemias at primary diagnosis (67 acute non-lymphoblastic leukemias = ANLL; 36 acute lymphoblastic or undifferentiated leukemias = ALL/AUL), 206 in complete remission (14 of them 1 to 2 months before a relapse was diagnosed clinically) and 60 at the diagnosis of relapse.

94 of 103 patients tested at primary diagnosis received intensive induction treatment: 62 patients with acute non-lymphoblastic leukemia were treated by EORTC-protocols containing adriamycin, vincristin and Ara-C; 32 patients with acute lymphoblastic or undifferentiated leukemia were treated within a study group in West-Germany by BMFT-protocols containing daunorubicin, vincristin, L-asparaginase and prednisone during the first phase and cyclophosphamide, Ara-C, methotrexate and 6-mercaptopurine during the second phase. In 59 patients (63%) a complete remission after induction treatment was achieved. 35 patients (37%) were non responder; that means in this representation treatment failure or partial remission.

Because of technical reasons not all parameters of the DNA metabolism could be performed in all marrow specimens. The corresponding numbers of evaluable results are given in those figures reporting the results. The methodolical steps are summarized in Figure 2.

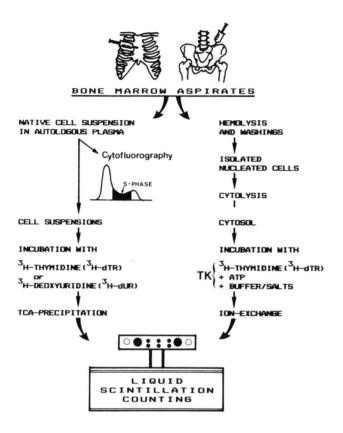

Figure 2. Determination of DNA synthesis
activities in human bone marrow cells:
Methods.

Nucleoside incorporation (25)

Without any further preparation, the bone
marrow specimens were adjusted with the patients
own serum to 10.000 and 20.000 nucleated cells
per microliter. Aliquots of 100 microliters of
these bone marrow cell suspensions were incubated
in triplicate in a water bath at 37°C with^{3}H-dTR
(10^{-5}M, 0,5 Ci/mmole) or ^{3}H-dUR(10^{-5}M, 0,5Ci/mmole).
The reaction was stopped by adding 1 ml ice-cold
saline (0,9% NaCl in water) after 1 hour.

To precipitate the acid insoluble material, which
contains the DNA, the complete cell suspension was
washed on a cellulose-acetate membrane filter
(Millipore HAWP 02500, 0,45 u) thrice with 2 ml 5%
trichloracetic acid and thrice with 2 ml 0,1 N
hydrochloric acid. Filters were dried, and the radioactivity was determined in a liquid scintillation
counter. Results of the nucleoside incorporation
into DNA were expressed in nmoles/min x 10^{10} nucleated cells.

Thymidine Kinase (TK) assay (26)

The erythrocytes of the bone marrow cell
suspension (see above) were lysed by 3 min incubation at $0°C$ with 5 ml 0,84% ammonium chloride.
The final count of nucleated cells was adjusted
to 100.000/ul with hypotonic 0.0007 M K-phosphate
buffer pH 7,4 after washing thrice with phosphate-
buffered saline. The debris of the lysed cells
were separated for the enzyme-containing supernatant by centrifugation (50.000 g, $4°C$) after an
incubation for 1 hour at $0°C$. TK assays were done
in triplicate: 100 ul of the supernatant were incubated with 100 ul of a substrate mixture containing 100 mM tris-buffer pH 8,0, 5 mM $MgCl_2$,
5 mM Mg-EDTA, 4,5 mM ATP and o,1 mM ^{3}H-dTR
(0.1 Ci/mmol). The reaction was stopped for 2 min
in a boiling water bath after 1 hour incubation in
a water bath at $37°C$. The assays were centrifugated
and 20 ul of the supernatant were transferred on
a DEAE-cellulose paper square (1 x 1 cm) and
washed twice for 10 min with 1 mM ammonium formate
solution, once for 5 min with water and once for
5 min with ethanol. The radioactivity was determined in a scintillation counter after drying.
TK activity was expressed in nmoles/min x 10^{10}
isolated nucleated bone marrow cells.

%S-phase cells (4)

The analysis of the cell cycle phases were
carried out with a Cytofluorograph 4800 A (Bio-
physics). The bone marrow cell suspension (see
above) were stained for DNA with propidiumiodide
(50 mg per 1000 ml 0,1% sodium-citrate solution)

for at least 15 min at 4°C. With a computer-assisted program, the DNA-histograms were analyzed and the relative contents of DNA-synthesizing cells in the bone marrow populations were expressed in %S.

Statistics

For comparing leukemic and normal bone marrow cells or remission versus no-remission, the Wilcoxon-test was used.

RESULTS AND DISCUSSION

Figure 3 summarizes the overall results of the DNA-synthesis activity in bone marrow specimens from patients with acute leukemia at primary diagnosis.

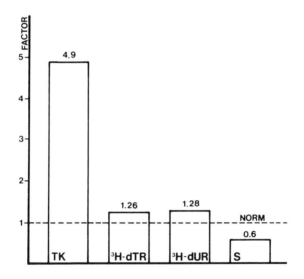

Figure 3. Parameters of DNA-synthesis in leukemic bone marrow cell populations at first diagnosis in comparison to normal bone marrow. Normal values are set to 1 for all parameters. Numbers of evaluable tests are: TK = 87, dTR = 41, dUR = 41, %S = 41.

Comparing the results from normal controls and
leukemic cells the activity of TK is increased by
a factor of 4,9 (p< 0.0001) in the latter. Much
smaller - at the border of significance (p < 0.05)
are the increased values of nucleoside incorporation-rates into intact leukemic bone marrow cells
having autologous conditions (patients own serum):
the factor is 1,26 for dTR and 1.28 for dUR. In
contrast to these findings the proportion of
S-phase cells in the leukemic cell population is
lower (factor 0,6; p <0.05). The sensitivity of
finding high TK-values in leukemic bone marrow
cells is 83%. The difference of TK-activity between normal and leukemic cells becomes even more
evident, if one calculates TK-activity in relation
to % S-phase cells in these populations. The ratio
TK/%S is increased in leukemias by a factor of
8,2. There is no difference between acute non-
lymphoblastic (ANLL) and acute lymphoblastic or
undifferentiated (ALL/AUL) leukemias in this
respect. Only 17% of the patients with acute
leukemia do not show a significantly increased
TK activity in their blast cells of the bone marrow.
Few of these patients even were characterized by
much lower TK-activity and also of the nucleoside
incorporation-rates compared to normal controls.
These cases are defined as "smoldering-leukemia".
They are not treated by intensive polychemotherapy,

       Thus, TK can be used as a sensitive marker
for rapid proliferating leukemias.

Figure 4 shows the changes of TK activity during
the course of acute leukemias. The high activity
at primary diagnosis is clearly reduced when
patients are in remission. But, statistically
it is still higher than in normal bone marrow
cells. However, in comparison to a factor of 4.9
at diagnosis, the factor during remission is
only 1.52. The TK activity during relapse reaches
again the same values as compared to the levels
seen at primary diagnosis. This increase of TK
becomes apparent 1 to 2 months before a relapse is
diagnosed clinically and by an new increase of
blast cells in the bone marrow.

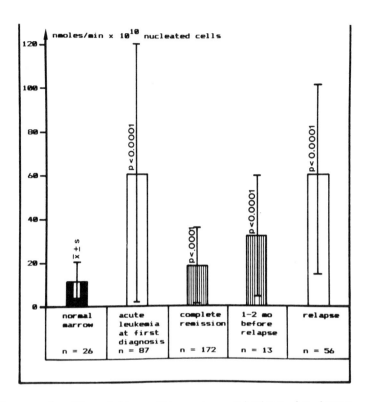

Figure 4. Thymidine Kinase activity in bone marrow cells of patients with acute leukemia at first diagnosis, in remission, and at relapse.

This phenomen is illustrated in more detail in Figure 5 presenting the course of two patients with acute leukemias. In case 1 after three months and in case 2 after two months of complete remission there is a sharp increase of TK activity at a time, when the blast count in the bone marrow is still as low as 7% resp. 6%.
Interestingly one month later a relapse of the acute leukemia is diagnosed by an increase of the blast counts in the bone marrow to 60% resp. 70%. Thus, the sharp increase of TK activity can occur earlier than the overt blastic transformation of the bone marrow.

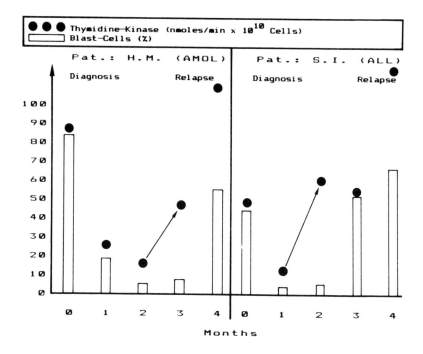

Figure 5. Thymidine kinase in bone marrow cells
as an early indicator for relapse of acute leukemias
= increase of thymidine kinase 1 month before
significant increase in bone marrow blast counts.

From these results it can be concluded that
serial measurements of TK during remission are
justified for controlling its quality. The per-
sistance of high TK-activity or a new increase can
predict relapse before a morphological diagnosis
in the bone marrow is possible.

Figure 6 shows the evaluation of the DNA-
synthesis in leukemic cells as prognostic indicator for predicting complete remission. Patients
who achieve complete remission after induction
treatment (adriamycin + vincristin + cytosine-
arabinoside for ANLL; daunorubicin + vincristin
+ L-asparaginase + prednisone for ALL/AUL)
(10,17) have lower activities for TK and nucleoside incorporations, but not for %S-phase cells. The
significance was only borderline for TK (p < 0.04),

but rather clear for the nucleoside incorporation
(p < 0.01). Thus, pretreatment TK-activity does not
predict the effect of intensive remission induction
treatment by polychemotherapy, although it is somewhat higher in patients who do not achieve complete
remission. Similarly, the nucleoside-incorporation-
rates (^{3}H-dTR and ^{3}H-dUR) into the DNA of leukemic
cells have only a minor potential of predicting
the treatment's outcome. Statistically the higher
DNA-synthesis activity seems to correlate with a
poor response, but because of the wide range of
standard deviations, a prediction cannot be made
for the individual patient.

 Pretreatment %S-phase-cells were not predictive for response in our patients. Similar results
were reported by others (9,21) when patients were
treated with anthracycline containing polychemotherapy regimens. If they were treated only with
antimetabolites (e.g. cytosine-arabinoside), a
higher %S-cells seemed to be correlated with more
complete remission (21).

 Another question was, whether early changes
in DNA-synthesis during the first three or four
days after the beginning of cytostatic treatment
can predict a therapeutic outcome. This analysis
is shown in Figure 7.

 Regarding biochemical changes in leukemic
cells during the first three to four days after
the beginning of treatment there is no effect of
TK-activity, but, nucleoside incorporation is inhibited more than 50%. As can be seen from these
preliminary results, there is no difference between patients who achieve complete remission and
those who do not. This is explained by the fact

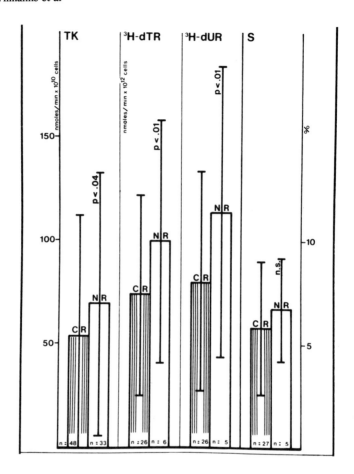

Figure 6. DNA synthesis in leukemic bone marrow
cell population: Pretreatment values and treatment
results after induction therapy.
CR = complete remission
NR = no complete remission

that the inhibition of DNA-synthesis may correspond
mainly to the cytoreduction in bone marrow, which
is observed in merely all treated patients and
which does not predict complete remission in all

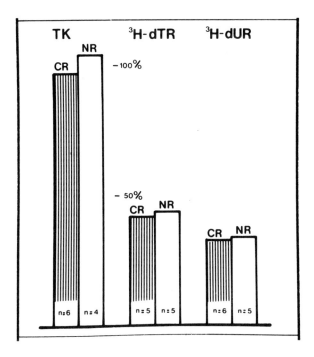

Figure 7. DNA-synthesis in leukemic bone marrow
cells: 3 or 4 days after the beginning of induction
therapy in comparison to pretreatment values (=100%).
CR = complete remission
NR = no complete remission.

cases. Further studies in a larger cohort of
patients are necessary to evaluate the question
whether biochemical parameters of the DNA-synthesis
at day 3 or 4 may have the same weight in predicting response as do quantitative cytology on day 6
(2) and cytokinetic data in bone marrow biopsies
(9) or aspirates (19) within the first week of
induction treatment, which are thought to predict
complete remission.

Ongoing investigations have to clarify whether there is a correlation between intracellular TK and serum TK (H.Sauer, in preparation).

SUMMARY

Selected key-steps in the biochemical path-ways of DNA-synthesis and cytokinetic parameters were measured in human bone marrow cells: Thymi-dine kinase (TK), incorporation of nucleosides (thymidine = dTR and deoxyuridine = dUR), % cells in DNA-synthesis-phase of the cell division cycle (%S). 26 normal marrow and a total of 369 marrow specimens from patients with acute leukemia were assayed either at first diagnosis, during remission, or at relapse. A significant 5-fold increase of TK was found in leukemic cells, thus, being a suitable marker for follow-up of these patients.

The sensitivity to detect a high TK at primary diagnosis of acute leukemia is 83%. An increase of TK during remission can indicate an imminent relapse before an increase of blast cells can be detected in the bone marrow. The incorporation-rates of dTR and dUR were also significantly in-creased in leukemic cells. Patients who did not achieve complete remission after induction treat-ment had higher incorporation-rates. In contrast to the enhanced biochemical activity of DNA-meta-bolism, %S-phase-cells were significant lower in leukemic cell populations. %S-phase cells did not correlate with treatment results.

An inhibition of DNA synthesis, estimated by the incorporation rates of dTR and dUR for more than 50% during the first 3-4 days after start of in-duction treatment corresponds with cytoreduction in the leukemic bone marrow which does not predict complete remission in all cases.

ACKNOWLEDGEMENTS

The authors express their thanks to P. Wetzl, B. Schwaier and V. Brumme for their skillful technical assistance. The study was supported by the Deutsche Forschungsgemeinschaft, AZ.: Wi 117/23 and by the Kind-Philipp-Foundation.

REFERENCES

1. Balley-Wood R, Dallimore CM, Smith SA, Whittaker JA (1984). Use of logistic regression analysis to improve prediction of prognosis in acute myeloid leukaemia. Leuk.Res. 8:667-681.
2. Barlogie B, Maddox AM, Johnston DA, Raber, MN, Dewinko B (1983). Quantitative cytology in leukemia research. Blood Cells 9: 35-56.
3. Bernard P, Reiffers J, Lacombe F, Dachary D, Boisseau MR, Broustet A (1984). A stage classification for prognosis in adult acute myelogenous leukemia based upon patient's age, bone marrow karyotypes and clinical features. Scand. J. Haematol. 32: 429-441.
4. Fleischer W, Pelka R (1978). A practical analysis of DNA-histograms with a laboratory computer. In Lutz D (ed.): Pulse Cytophotometry. European Press, Ghent/Belgium: pp 137-143.
5. Freireich EJ (1983). Methods for evaluating response to treatment in adult acute leukemia. Blood Cells 9: 5-20.
6. French M, Byron PA, Fiere D, Vuvan H, Guyotat D (1986). Cell-Cycle prognostic value in adult acute myeloid leukemia. The choice of the best variables. Leuk.Res. 10: 51-58.
7. Gustavsson A, Olofsson T (1984). Prediction of response to chemotherapy in acute leukemia by in vitro drug sensitivity testing on leukemic stem cells. Cancer Res. 44: 4648-4653.
8. Hagberg H, Gronowitz S, Killander A, Källander C, Simonsson B, Sundström C, Öberg G (1984). Serum thymidine kinase in acute leukaemia. Br.J. Cancer 49: 537-540.
9. Hiddemann W, Büchner T, Andreeff M, Wörmann E, Melamed MR, Clarkson BD (1982). Cellkinetics

in acute leukemia. A critical reevaluation
based on new data. Cancer 50:250-258.
10. Hoelzer D,Thiel E, Löffler H, Bodenstein H,
Plaumann L (1984). Intensified therapy in
acute lymphoblastic and acute undifferentiated leukemia in adults.Blood 64: 38-47.
11. Hörnstein P, Lindquist R, Gahrton G (1984).
Prognostic implications of in vitro colony
and clonal chromosomal aberrations in adults
with acute leukemia. Scand.J.Haematol 32:
297-306.
12. Hofman V, Berens ME(1984). Test this patients
leukemic stem cell in a non-clonogenic
chemosensitivity assay. Treat according to
standard protocols. Eur. J. Cancer Clin.
Oncol. 20: 1119-1123.
13. Hutton JJ, Coleman MS, Mofitt S, Greenwood MF,
Holland P (1982). Prognostic significance of
therminal transferase activity in childhood
acute lymphoblastic leukemia: a prospective
analysis of 164 patients. Blood 60:1267-1276.
14. Jehn U, Wachholz K (1983). Kinetics of colony-
forming cells (CFU-c) in adult acute leukemia and their prognostic relevance.
Leuk. Res. 7: 761-770.
15. Jehn U, Kern D, Wachholz K, Hoelzel D (1983).
Prognostic value of in vitro growth pattern
of colony forming cells in adult acute leukemia. Brit.J.Cancer 47: 423-428.
16. Jehn U, Wachholz K (1985). CFU-gm colony formation of peripheral blood and bone marrow
in adult acute leukemia at presentation,
during remission, and at a relapse. Inter J.
Cell Cloning 3: 199-213.
17. Jehn U, Zittoun R (1985). AML-6-Studie zum
Wert einer zyklischen alternierenden Chemo-
therapie während der Remission bei akuter
myeloischer Leukämie. Onkologie 8: 94-96.
18. Look AT, Roberson PK,Williams DL, Rivera G,
Bowman WP, Pui CH (1985). Prognostic importance of blast cell DNA content in childhood acute lymphoblastic leukemia. Blood 65:
1079-1086.
19. Murphy SB, Dahl GV, George SL, Karas J,
Look AT (1982). Determination of the signi-

ficance of in vitro blast cell (3H)-thymidine labelling indices obtained initially and serially during therapy of acute non-lymphoblastic leukemia. Leuk.Res. 6:639-648.

20. Preisler HD , Reese PA, Marinello MJ, Pothier L (1983). Adverse effects of aneuploidy on the outcome of remission induction for acute non-lymphocytic leukemia: analysis of types of treatment failure. Brit. J. Haematol. 53: 459-466.

21. Preisler HD, Azarnia N, Raza A, Grunwald H, Vogler R (1984). Relationship between the per cent of marrow cells in S phase and the outcome of remission induction therapy for acute nonlymphocytic leukaemia. Brit. J. Haematol. 56: 399-408.

22. Preisler HD, Azarnia N, Marinello M (1984). Relationship of the growth of leukemic cells in vitro to the outcome of therapy for acute nonlymphocytic leukemia. Cancer Res. 44: 1718-1725.

23. Preisler HD, Epstein J, Raza A, Azarnia N, Browman G (1984). Inhibition of DNA synthesis by cytosine arabinoside - Relation to response of acute non-lymphocytic leukemia to remission induction therapy and stage of disease. Eur.J. Cancer Clin. Oncol. 20: 1061-1069.

24. Pui CH, Dodge RK, Dahl GV, Rivera G, Look AT, Klawinsky D (1985). Serum lactic dehydrogenase level has prognostic value in childhood acute lymphoblastic leukemia. Blood 66:778-782.

25. Sauer H, Wilmanns W (1977). Cobalamin dependent methionine synthesis and methyl-folate-trap in human vitamin B12 deficiency. Brit.J. Haematol. 36: 189-198.

26. Sauer H, Wilmanns W (1983). Thymidine kinase. ATP: thymidine 5'-phosphotransferase, EC 2.7.1.21. In Bergmeyer HU (ed.): Methods of Enzymatic Analysis. Verlag Chemie, Weinheim/West-Germany, Vol.III: pp 468-474.

27. Scavennec J, Cailla H, Gastaut JA, Maraninchi D, Carcassonne Y (1982). 2' - and 3' -ribonucleoside monophosphate in leukocytes of acute myeloid leukemia: markers for early diagnosis of relapse. Int. J. Cancer 29: 257-259.

28. Schwartz RS, Mackintosh FR, Halpern J, Schreir SL, Greenberg PL (1984). Multivariant analysis of factors associated with outcome of treatment for adults with acute myelogenous leukemia. Cancer 54: 1672-1681.

29. Schwarzmeier JD, Paietta E, Mittermayer K, Pirker R (1984). Prediction of the response to chemotherapy in acute leukemia by short-term test in vitro. Cancer 53: 390-395.

30. Shen BJ, Ekert H, Tauro GP, Bladeras A (1984). Left shift in peripheral blood count at diagnosis in acute lymphocytic leukemia is significantly correlated with duration of complete remission. Blood 63: 216-219.

31. Wilmanns W (1971). DNA-synthesis in leukemic cells under the action of cytotoxic agents in vitro and in vivo. In Hall TC (ed.): Prediction of Response in Cancer Therapy, Nat.Cancer Institute Monograph 34; pp. 153-159.

32. Wilmanns W, Wilms K (1972). DNA-Synthesis in normal and leukemic cells as related to therapy with cytotoxic drugs. Enzyme 13: 90-98.

33. Wilmanns W, Sauer H, Wilms K (1975). Untersuchungen der DNS-Synthese als Grundlage für eine rationale Kombinationsbehandlung bei akuten Leukämien. In Vogt W, Bock HE (eds.): Klinische Pharmakologie und experimentelle Therapie. Editio Cantor Aulendorf/West Germany: pp 3-19.

34. Yunis JJ, Brunning RD, Howe RB, Lobell M (1984). High-resolution chromosomes as an independent indicator in adult acute non-lymphocytic leukemia. N. Engl. J. Med. 311: 812-819.

35. Zittoun R, Cadiou M, Bayle C, Suciu S, Solbu G, Hayat M (1984). Prognostic value of cytologic parameters in acute myelogenous leukemia. Cancer 53: 1526-1532.

Prediction of Response to Cancer Therapy, pages 255–264
© 1988 Alan R. Liss, Inc.

THE EORTC CLONOGENIC ASSAY SCREENING STUDY GROUP (CASSG)
PROGRAM

Matti S. Aapro, for J.F. Eliason, C. Herman,
M. Uitendaal, M. Rozencweig and members of the
CASSG

Division d'Onco-Hématologie, Hôpital Cantonal
Universitaire, 1211 Geneva 4, Switzerland

INTRODUCTION

The European Organization for Research and Treatment
of Cancer has several cooperative groups which study new
drugs for cancer treatment. Among these, the Clonogenic
Assay Screening Study Group (CASSG) was founded in 1981
with the following aims.

TABLE 1. CASSG
favors

---

1) rapid dissemination of data in order to standardize
   methods of tumor growth and drug testing in vitro

2) free exchange of ideas between clinicians and cell
   biologists, pharmacologists, etc.

3) prospective studies in association with clinical EORTC
   protocols to test the clinical or biologic significance
   of in vitro tumor study techniques

4) collaborative in vitro phase I (bone marrow toxicity)
   and phase II (fresh tumor samples) studies testing drugs
   and drug combinations

The group is open to all investigators interested in
clinical and biological aspects of tumor cell growth in

vitro. It is presently comprised of laboratories in nine European countries (Austria, Belgium, Denmark, France, Germany, Great-Britain, Italy, Netherlands, Switzerland). This article should present the philosophy of the group's work, some of its results and a perspective for its possible role in the EORTC.

FIRST GENERATION WiDr STUDY

Colony forming cell assays are one of many methods to evaluate the biology of tumor cells. They exploit the capability of transformed cells to grow in vitro in a semisolid medium (methylcellulose, agarose, agar). This property is shared by most transformed cells, and colonies may be representative of the progenitor cells that perpetuate a tumor in vivo. Several techniques are available (Courtenay, 1978; Salmon, 1978; Eliason, 1984), and they all share some basic principles.

TABLE 2. BASIC PRINCIPLES OF COLONY FORMING CELL ASSAYS

Obtain a fresh tumor sample

Transform into a single cell suspension

Put into semi-solid medium, 37°C,
    air/CO_2 or low oxygen/CO_2 atmosphere

Evaluate "clumps" at day 1

Evaluate growth of colonies days 14 to 28
in presence or absence of other agents

This apparently simple procedure hides a variety of technical and theoretical problems, evident to all investigators. Unfortunately these problems were not always recognized (Selby, 1982).

The CASSG decided, as one of its first goals, to assure QUALITY CONTROL for the work of participating European laboratories. A first study was designed to establish the interlaboratory reproducibility of in vitro cell growth and drug sensitivity findings. All participants were supplied with the same batch of a colon carcinoma cell line (WiDr, ATCC CCL 218). It became evident that the plating efficiency of the cell line was highly dependent upon the exact medium used in different laboratories and on the way it was passaged. Therefore it was not surprising that drug testing was not reproducible, as some major quality control check points were not assured (Rozencweig, 1983).

The Southwest Oncology Group (SWOG) and the Southeastern Cancer Study Group (SECSG) had also decided to evaluate the reproducibility of these colony assays (Clark, 1984; Luedke, 1984). The SWOG study was similar to the CASSG one, in that a cell line was shipped to all participating centers, whereas the SECSG shipped samples containing minced SOTO tumor (a xenograft grown in athymic mice). This latter approach is interesting, in that it more closely resembles to the situation of fresh human solid tumor samples. Both groups had considerable problems with variable growth, large coefficients of variation in some experiments and some drugs that could not be tested adequately.

SECOND GENERATION WiDr STUDY

Subsequently the CASSG decided to standardize the assay methodology in participating laboratories. This attempt proved to be impossible, in that the commercial suppliers could not assure delivery of the same batches of material all over Europe. However, in spite of this shortcoming, study 37841 provided very interesting data.

One can observe in table 3 that our positive control, sodium azide, and 5-fluorouracil (at high concentrations) were tested satisfactorily by the majority of centers. Bleomycin however could not be tested in a reproducible way, in that there was considerable disagreement between laboratories about its effect at 10 ug/ml. One reason is that this concentration is very similar to the 50% inhibitory concentration for this cell line, and one is thus testing the steep portion of the dose-response curve, where minor changes in drug concentration or cell sensitivity can have major influence on the number of observed colonies. Another reason is that the linearity of colony growth was not always assured, and this may be an important factor in the reliability of percentage colony survival data.

This study was the basis for an important observation concerning sodium azide : when Petri dishes containing 6 mg/ml of sodium azide were placed together with cultures of WiDr cells in a large Petri dish and incubated at 37°C in an atmosphere of 10% CO_2/air, no growth could be observed. Colonies were formed only in cultures separated from the sodium azide dishes, with an inverse relationship to the distance of the test cultures from the azide treated plates. It is probable that hydrazaic acid, a highly toxic vapour, is responsible of this phenomenon (Lelieveld, 1986).

TABLE 3. PREDICTION OF RESISTANCE PROFILES

study 37841

INTERLABORATORY DATA

M. Uitendaal, study chairman

PURPOSE : cell line (colon, WiDr) tested simultaneously in several laboratories : Evaluation of colony survival should be the same.

DRUG	number of tests	<30% survival	30-60% survival	>60% survival
AZIDE				
60 ug/ml	9	7	1	1
600 ug/ml	9	9	0	0
5-FU				
30 ug/ml	10	10	0	0
300 ug/ml	10	10	0	0
BLEOMYCIN				
10 ug/ml	10	2	3	5
100 ug/ml	10	8	2	0

BI-ANNUAL QUALITY CONTROL (37851, 37861, 37871)

The group decided that fully standardized techniques were impossible to achieve without considerable funding for technical assistance. One has to realize that each laboratory uses its culture system for different purposes which make it difficult to use a "standard" system. It was therefore felt that a standardized cell line could be used to compare the results obtained with the different systems.

WiDr cells are mailed as viable, proliferating cells, to all participating laboratories. Cell concentrations, times for passaging the cells, in a centrally supplied standard medium, and specific counting parameters are strictly defined. A total of 15 laboratories participated in both runs of the first study.

TABLE 4. QUALITY CONTROL STUDY 37851
          J. Eliason, study chairman

number laboratories	linearity	suboptimal growth
15	29/32 tests	14/32 tests

Linearity is a major concern for our group, as already stated. From the figure below one can easily understand that a decrease of the observed colony number from 2 y to y may represent quite different decreases in the actual number of killed progenitor cells, depending on the type of relationship between the number of cells plated and the number of colonies. Non-linearity has to be looked for when one does studies with cell lines or fresh human tumor samples (Meyskens, 1983; Eliason, 1985). It is therefore very satisfactory to observe that, provided one plates WiDr cells in adequate concentrations, the group as a whole provides data with a linear relationship between cells plated and number of observed colonies. However, suboptimal growth was observed in many centers, probably due to damage to cells during shipment.

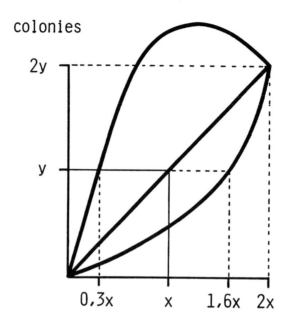

Figure 1. Possible relationships between number of cells plated and colonies observed.

Based on these encouraging data the CASSG ran two quality control studies in 1986. They were designed in the same way as the previous study, only that abrin, cisplatin and doxorubicin were tested by all laboratories, in addition to linearity studies.

Figure 2 shows the dose-response curve of WiDr to doxorubicin and indicates that the group as a whole performed very satisfactorily. We can see that run Ia-1 of the study, done in the spring, gives the same dose-response curve for doxorubicin as the later (fall) run Ia-2. The error bars represent the standard deviation of the curves, which are computed from the results reported by the participating investigators.

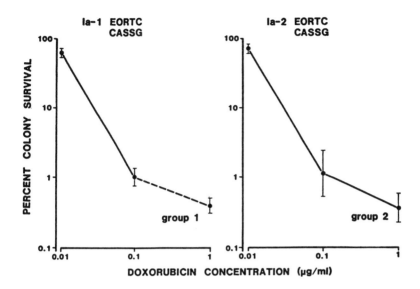

Figure 2. Dose-response curve of WiDr to doxorubicin

In 1987 two further studies, with different drugs, will be run. Altogether these 3 studies will form the basis of our continued quality control studies and should allow the group to represent another reliable system for drug screening in Europe.

CISPLATIN ANALOGUE STUDY (37842)

One of the aims of the group is to provide clinically relevant indications in drug screening. A first trial has been a study run in 1985 which acquired 114 fresh human tumor samples within 4 months and was designed to evaluate cisplatin, carboplatin (paraplatin[R]) and iproplatin.

Table 5 shows that one needs an in vitro concentration of 10 times that of cisplatin in order to achieve a similar reduction in the number of colonies with the other agents. Although the study hasn't been fully analyzed, it appears that the activity of cisplatin and its derivatives is similar, i.e. there is a pattern of in vitro cross-resistance.

TABLE 5. CISPLATIN ANALOGUE STUDY

study 37842

OVARIAN TUMORS

C. Herman, study chairman

ONE HOUR EXPOSURE TO DRUG

	concentrations (ug/ml)	samples with >50% colony reduction
CISPLATIN	0.1	23 %
	1.0	64 %
CARBOPLATIN	1	14 %
	10	50 %
IPROPLATIN	1	25 %
	10	46 %

The CASSG should be able to continue similar studies, in parallel to phase II studies run by other EORTC cooperative groups. Even though there are considerable data that point to the clinical usefulness of such an approach, we caution that it will not be possible to rely on our in vitro system before several such prospective parallel studies are run.

FUTURE STUDIES

The CASSG is presently evaluating the capability of its members to maintain several cell lines and test them against standard agents (doxorubicin, cisplatin, VP-16, melphalan) in a reproducible way. This will form the basis for comparative studies with new agents, which should begin in 1988.

CONCLUSION

Our group has established a network of collaborating centers in Europe, with expertise in the field of cell culture and several other techniques that can be used for drug sensitivity testing. We have shown that drug data can be provided on a very reliable basis by the group, and will continue to assure this quality control, which may include other assays, e.g. DNA precursor uptake tests. Table 6 describes the way in which our group might be used for the study of a new compound (drug X). This system is not as complex and by no means as expensive as that of the U.S. National Cancer Institute (described in this volume), but might represent a complement, in that it is not aimed at primary screening, but should confirm the activity of a compound and define its target tumors.

TABLE 6. POSSIBLE ROLE(S) OF THE CASSG

	MAXIMAL CONCENTRATION IN BONE MARROW (CONTINUOUS EXPOSURE)	CELL LINES**	ASSAY TYPE	PROFILE OF CELL LINE AND BONE MARROW ACTIVITY (COMPARED TO "REFERENCE" AGENTS)	EXTENSIVE TESTING (SCHEDULE DEPENDENCY ANALOGUE COMPARISON)
SOLUTION OF DRUG X*		BREAST	- COLONY FORMATION		FRESH TUMOR SAMPLE VALIDATION (IN VITRO PHASE II)
		KIDNEY	- DYE EXCLUSION		
VEHICLE CONTROL		OVARY	- CROSS-CHECKING BY USE OF SOME CELL- LINES IN 2 OR MORE LABORATORIES		XENOGRAFT EVALUATION (WITHIN AND OUTSIDE GROUP)
		MELANOMA			
		LUNG (SC & NSC)			
		BRAIN			
		COLON			
		HEAD, NECK			

* KNOWN TO BE ACTIVE

** ALSO CHARACTERIZED FOR SENSITIVITY TO "REFERENCE" ACTIVE AND FALSELY ACTIVE AGENTS (DRUGS, HORMONES) DIFFERENT FROM NCI CELL LINES

ANTIMETABOLITES, DRUGS REQUIRING ACTIVATION: SPECIAL PROCEDURES

REFERENCES

Clark GM, von Hoff DD (1984). Quality control of a multi-
center human tumor cloning system: The Southwest Oncology
Group experience. In: Salmon SE and Trent JM (eds):
"Human Tumor Cloning," Orlando: Grune & Stratton, pp 255-
265.
Courtenay VD, Selby PJ, Smith IE, Mills J, Peckham MJ
(1978). Growth of human tumor cell colonies from biopsies
using two-soft agar techniques. Br J Cancer 38:77-81.
Eliason JF, Fekete A, Odartchenko N (1984). Improving
techniques for clonogenic assays. Recent Res Cancer Res
94:267-275.
Eliason JF, Aapro MS, Decrey D, Brink-Petersen M (1985).
Non-linearity of colony formation by human tumour cells
from biopsy samples. Br J Cancer 52:311-318.
Lilieveld P, Aapro MS, van Lambalgen R, van der Berg KJ
(1986). Sodium azide is less suitable as a positive control of drug-induced lethality for in vitro clonogenic
assays. Invest New Drugs 4:367-371.
Luedke DW, Carey FJ, Krishan A, Chee D, Chang B, Franco R,
Niell HB, Johns ME, Kenady DE, Zirvi K (1984). Interlaboratory reproducibility of the human tumor colony forming
assay (HTCA): The Southeastern Cancer Study Group (SECSG)
experience. In: Salmon SE and Trent JM (eds): "Human
Tumor Cloning", Orlando: Grune & Stratton, pp 245-254.
Meyskens FL, Thompson SP, Hickie RA, Sipes NJ (1983).
Potential biological explanation of stimulation of colony
growth in semi-solid agar by cytotoxic agents. Br J
Cancer 48:863-868.
Rozencweig M (1983). Quality control study of the human
tumor clonogenic assay. Proceedings AACR 24:313.
Salmon SE, Hamburger AW, Soehnlen B, Curie BGM, Alberts DS,
Moon TE (1978). Quantitation of differential sensitivity
of human tumor stem cells to anticancer drugs. N Engl J
Med 298:1321-1327.
Selby P, Buick N, Tannock I (1982). A critical appraisal of
the "human stem cell assay". N Engl J Med 308:129-134.

Prediction of Response to Cancer Therapy, pages 265–286
© 1988 Alan R. Liss, Inc.

DEVELOPMENT OF HUMAN TUMOR CELL LINE PANELS FOR USE IN
DISEASE-ORIENTED DRUG SCREENING

Robert H. Shoemaker, Anne Monks*, Michael C.
Alley, Dominic A. Scudiero*, Donald L. Fine*,
Theodore L. McLemore, Betty J. Abbott, Kenneth
D. Paull, Joseph G. Mayo, and Michael R. Boyd

Developmental Therapeutics Program, Division of
Cancer Treatment, National Cancer Institute,
Bethesda, MD 20892, U.S.A. and *Program Resources
Inc., National Cancer Institute-Frederick Cancer
Research Facility, Frederick, MD 21701, U.S.A.

INTRODUCTION

The potential value of in vitro drug sensitivity assays
as predictors of clinical response in individual patients
has been limited by technical difficulties in obtaining,
handling, culturing and assaying tumor samples [1-6] and by
the lack of clinically effective drugs for the common adult
solid tumors [7,8], especially lung and colon carcinoma.
While studies have indicated potential predictive value for
soft agar colony forming assays [3,9-18] as well as for
other types of in vitro assays [19-21] the practical utility
of these assays to clinical oncologists will remain limited
until more effective drugs are available.

As an approach to discovery of new compounds for
possible clinical evaluation against particular tumor types,
we are investigating the use of disease-oriented panels of
human tumor cell lines for large-scale drug screening [22,
23]. This approach differs in several fundamental ways
from antitumor drug screening models used previously by the
National Cancer Institute and other investigators. In
previous approaches, primary drug screening employed in
vivo models and relied on only one, or a few transplantable
tumors (generally murine leukemias L1210 or P388). The in
vitro based model which we are developing for the new
primary screen will employ large numbers of human tumor cell

lines organized into disease-oriented panels representative
of several of the major human malignancies. Each compound
will be tested in every cell line in the screening panels.
In this screening strategy compounds are sought which
selectively inhibit the growth of particular cell types
within the disease-oriented cell line panels. Such compounds will then be further evaluated in vivo using nude
mouse xenograft models against the appropriate tumor cell
lines from the in vitro primary screening panels [24].
In order to enhance the probability of identifying unique
compounds it is critical to maintain a large screening
capacity with the new model. We have, therefore, developed
methods consistent with screening at rates comparable to or
greater than previous in vivo screens operated by the
National Cancer Institute, i.e. 10,000 test materials per
year. In this report we will describe the current status
of this new in vitro based, disease-oriented drug screening
model with emphasis on development of the cell line panels,
implementation of automated assay methodology, and feasibility of the model for large-scale screening.

DEVELOPMENT OF CELL LINE PANELS

Since the mid-1950's, a large number of human tumor
cell lines have been established. However, certain tumor
types have been substantially more difficult to grow than
others. Initially, we have established pilot screening
panels representing carcinomas of the lung, colon, ovary,
and kidney; melanoma; central nervous system malignancies;
leukemia; and a miscellaneous panel which includes cell
lines with acquired multidrug resistance. Over 100 cell
lines, have been acquired, expanded in culture, evaluated
for the presence of adventitious agents (mycoplasma and
pathogenic mouse viruses), and cryopreserved. A subset of
these were adapted to growth in a standard culture medium
(RPMI 1640 supplemented with ten percent fetal bovine serum
and 2 mM L-glutamine) and further characterized to verify
human origin (isoenzyme studies and karyology), production
of tumors in nude mice of appropriate histology, and suita-
bility for use with the assay methodology to be employed.
The initial selection of cell lines for the screening panels
has been based on several considerations including: 1.
Utilization of multiple cell lines for each tumor type.

2. Employment of representatives of major histologic subtypes. 3. Utilization of cell lines which retain appropriate features of the tumor of origin. The initial screening panel thus derived is shown in Table 1. It should be emphasized that this represents a preliminary selection of lines for use in further refinement of the screening model and for pilot-scale screening studies. The final selection of cell lines to be employed in the full-scale implementation of the new screen may include some or all of the current lines as well as an appropriate additional selection of lines as available.

Lung Cancer

Because of the diversity of histologic subtypes observed in human lung cancer a relatively large proportion of the tumor cell lines in our initial screening panel are of this category. Ten non-small cell lung cancer cell lines representing squamous, adenosquamous, adenocarcinoma, bronchioloalveolar carcinoma, and large cell carcinoma have been included. Five small cell lung cancer cell lines representing the "classic" and "variant" forms described by Minna et al. and a line which differs from these in that it grows as an attached cell population in culture (DMS-114) are currently being utilized. These lung cancer cell lines produce subcutaneous tumors in nude mice with histology corresponding to the tumor cell lines. Striking growth has been observed following intrabronchial instillation of these cells, enabling use of an in vivo assay for follow-up testing of screening leads in which the tumor distribution, microenvironment, etc. may correspond more closely to that observed in the clinic. In this intrabronchial model, tumor progression can be monitored by noninvasive roentgenographic techniques [55].

Many of the lung cancer lines demonstrate a high degree of heterogeneity in their morphologic appearance and in their growth rates/kinetics. In several cases, e.g. NCI-H23, a marked degree of morphologic heterogeneity is observed within the cell population following plating at clonal density. Representation and preservation of some of the heterogeneity known to exist in lung cancer has been a major consideration in development of the lung cancer screening panel.

Colon Cancer

The composition of the current colon cancer cell line
panel includes four well known and widely used lines and one
relatively new line established in the laboratory of Dr.
Isiah Fidler (HCC 2998). All lines produce detectable levels
of carcinoembryonic antigen and form adenocarcinomas in nude
mice.

Ovarian Cancer

The current ovarian carcinoma cell line panel consists of
a series of "OVCAR" lines established recently by Drs. Thomas
Hamilton and Robert Ozols and one older line (A2780). Two of
the lines (OVCAR-5 and A2780) are from untreated patients and
the remainder are from patients who have undergone combination
chemotherapy. All the lines produce adenocarcinomas following
subcutaneous injection into nude mice. The OVCAR-3 line is
particularly useful for _in vivo_ therapeutic studies as it
produces a lethal intraabdominal carcinomatosis following
intraperitoneal injection in nude mice.

Renal Cancer

Three long established lines, A498, A704, and Caki-1 and
two new renal cancer lines, SN-12K1 and UO-31 are included in
our current panel. All produce adenocarcinomas in nude mice.

Melanoma

Four out of five of the melanoma lines in the panel
reportedly produce melanin. The amelanotic LOX line was
derived from a metastatic lesion in a patient with melanoma
and was included to represent this frequent clinical variant.
The LOX line retains metastatic ability in nude mice and has
served as the basis for the first practical metastatic model
of human cancer in nude mice for therapeutic studies [56].

Brain Tumors

The current brain tumor panel consists of four glioblastoma lines and a single medulloblastoma line (Te-671).
This latter line as well as the U-251 glioblastoma have
proven useful for _in vivo_ chemotherapeutic studies in nude

mice as intracranial models [57]. The "SNB" lines are relatively new ones established in the laboratory of Dr. Paul Kornblith.

Leukemia

Two lymphoid and two myeloid leukemia lines are included in the current panel. MOLT-4 and CEM were both derived from patients with common acute leukemia (cALL). Expression of CD4 receptors and terminal deoxynucleotidyl transferase support characterization of these as T lymphocyte derived neoplasms. The K562 line was established from a patient with chronic myelogenous leukemia and has been shown to differentiate along erythroid, myeloid, and monocytic pathways. The HL-60 promyelocytic leukemia line has been widely used for in vitro studies of "differentiating" agents.

Miscellaneous Panel

The phenomenon of multidrug resistance (MDR) has been increasingly studied in recent years and seems likely to be one of the factors which limits the effectiveness of existing chemotherapy [58]. In order to explore this phenomenon in a drug screening mode, the MCF-7 human breast cancer line and an MDR variant selected by in vitro treatment with adriamycin (the MCF-7/ADR line) and P388 murine leukemia and an MDR variant selected by in vivo treatment with adriamycin (the P388/ADR line) have been included in the current screening panels. These pairs of wild type/MDR lines may provide the potential for identifying agents with particular activity against MDR cell populations.

ASSAY DEVELOPMENT

As mentioned above, a key element in the current screening strategy is to maintain capacity for high volume screening. Considering a screening panel of 50 cell lines and an annual throughput of 10,000 compounds, the magnitude of the laboratory task can be computed as: (50 cell lines) (5 test concentrations) (duplicate cultures) (10,000 compounds/year) = 5 million cultures/year. The magnitude of this task dictates that any proposed assay methodology employ micro-

scale cultures, technical simplicity, speed, and
potential for automation. We have considered and evaluated
several assays which could potentially meet these requirements. The most promising of these appears to be a colormetric
growth inhibition assay which is based on metabolic reduction
of a tetrazolium salt to a colored formazan inside viable
cells. While this phenomenon has been long utilized in
histochemical procedures [59-61] and in some of the earliest
work on in vitro antitumor drug sensitivity testing [62], it
has only recently been employed for viability determinations
in association with growth inhibition assays. Mosmann [63]
has established that under appropriate conditions a linear
relationship is obtained between viable cell number and
formazan optical density measured using a standard Elisa
plate reader. We [64] and others [65,66] have evaluated
the application of this technology to anticancer drug
sensitivity testing and have found the method to be accurate
and highly reproducible. We have recently reported development of a new tetrazolium reagent (XTT) which produces a
water soluble formazan rather than the insoluble formazan
generated by classic tetrazolium reagents [67]. This
development has allowed further simplification of the
microculture tetrazolium assay as illustrated in Figure 1.

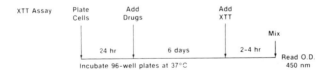

Figure 1. Simplified microculture tetrazolium
assay protocol using XTT for production of
water soluble formazan.

Cells are plated in 96-well microculture plates, incubated
for 24 hours, drugs (or appropriate control treatments) are
then added to each drugs well, the plates are incubated for
an additional six days, 50 μl of XTT solution is then added
to each well, the plates are incubated for an additional 4-6
hours, after brief mixing on a plate mixer, XTT formazan

optical density is measured at 450 nm using an Elisa reader
interfaced to a microcomputer based data processing system.

OPERATIONAL RESULTS IN PILOT-SCALE SCREENING

Utilizing the cell line panels shown in Table 1 and the
methods described above, a series of pilot-scale screening
studies have been performed. These screening studies have
included compounds with established clinical activity,
compounds identified in previous in vivo based screens which
have proven inactive in clinical trials, compounds currently
under consideration for development, as well as several
categories of "unknown" compounds. More than 45,000 dose-
response assays involving several hundred compounds have
been amassed in the computer data base. Reproducibility of
assay results has been monitored prospectively through the
use of a standard series of adriamycin dilutions which have
been tested on each occasion an individual cell line is used
for screening (weekly). No evidence for systematic drift in
sensitivity has been observed over the passage interval
utilized (20 serial passages).

Available screening results clearly indicate that individual cell lines show characteristic degrees of in vitro
chemosensitivity and unique responses to individual test
compounds. Examination of the overall patterns of sensitivity for the cell lines in the current disease-oriented
screening panels shows some associations with patterns of
clinical chemosensitivity. Figure 2 illustrates this
phenomen by ranking the sensitivity of cell lines based on
the percentage of times the line showed an IC_{50} (concentration resulting in 50% growth inhibition) for an individual
test compound which was one log or more lower than the
overall average IC_{50} for all cell lines tested against
that compound. Probably the most striking feature of this
analysis is the relative sensitivity of the leukemia and
small cell lung cancer lines. This result seems consistent
with the origin of the majority of the compounds tested in
preclinical drug development programs based on murine
leukemia models. Renal tumors showed overall resistance
and non-small cell lung cancer lines showed marked heterogeneity of response. It should be noted that these
associations with clinical chemosensitivity have been

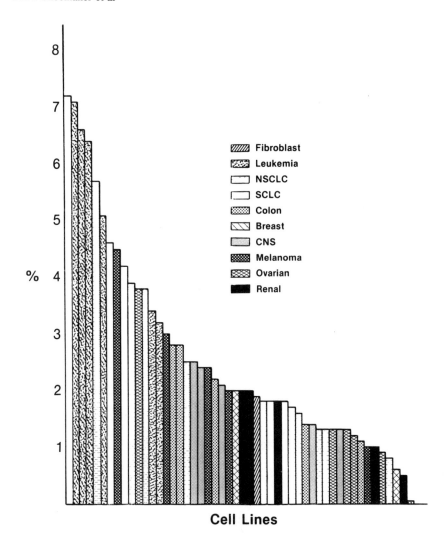

Figure 2. Relative cell line sensitivities of disease types estimated by the percentage of times log IC_{50} is at least one log more potent than the mean IC_{50}.

observed in cell lines which were not selected on the basis of their in vitro sensitivity to established agents. The "correlation" with clinical activity patterns could potentially be increased by engineering the individual cell line panels, replacing sensitive or resistant cell lines to obtain a desired balance. We have avoided this practice on the premise that this type of "calibration" procedure may engineer out of the model the potential for identifying entirely new types of agents with mechanisms of action which are not represented among currently available drugs.

In spite of this lack of selection of cell lines, unique and reproducible patterns of sensitivity of cell lines to well known drugs were observed which have associations with clinical patterns of activity. Examples of this are presented in Figures 3 and 4, for BCNU and bleomycin respectively.

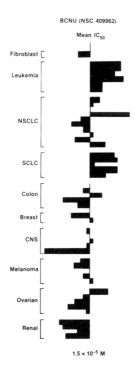

Figure 3. Pattern of sensitivity of disease-oriented cell line panels to BCNU. Responses to the right of the mean IC_{50} line (1.5×10^{-5} M) are more sensitive than the mean, while those on the left are more resistant.

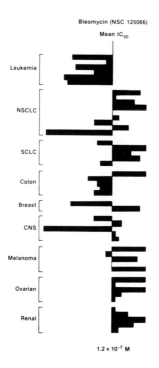

Figure 4. Pattern of sensitivity of disease-oriented
cell line panels to bleomycin. Responses to the right
of the mean IC_{50} line (1.2×10^{-7}M) are more sensitive
than the mean, while those on the left are more resistant.

In each case, a broad range of response, as measured by the
IC_{50} values, was observed. In the case of BCNU, as for
several other established agents, the leukemia and small
cell lung cancer lines showed consistent sensitivity.
Renal and colon carcinoma lines were relatively resistant.
However, as indicated by the results for bleomycin, this was
not invariably the case. Leukemia lines were quite resistant
to bleomycin and the renal lines relatively sensitive. Many
other examples are available which demonstrate "fingerprints"
of cell line sensitivity to individual agents. In several
instances similar fingerprints are observed for mechanistically
related compounds i.e., alkylating agents, DNA binders, etc.

TABLE 1

COMPOSITION OF INITIAL
DISEASE-ORIENTED SCREENING PANELS

Histology Cell Line	Institution (Source*)	Reference	Prior Chemotherapy**
NON-SMALL CELL LUNG CANCER			
<u>Adenocarcinoma</u>			
A549/Asc-1	National Cancer Institute (NCI-TB)	25	Unknown
EKVX	Norsk Hydro's Institute Oslo, Norway (O. Fodstad)	-	Unknown
NCI-H23	National Cancer Institute (A.F. Gazdar)	26,27	No
NCI-H522	National Cancer Insitute (A.F. Gazdar)	28	No
<u>Adeno-Squamous Carcinoma</u>			
NCI-H125	National Cancer Institute (A.F. Gazdar)	27,28	No
<u>Squamous Cell Carcinoma</u>			
NCI-H520	National Cancer Institute (A.F. Gazdar)	27,28,29	No
SK-MES-1	Memorial Sloan-Kettering Cancer Center (ATCC)	30	Unknown
<u>Bronchiolo-Alveolar Carcinoma</u>			
NCI-H322	National Cancer Institute (A.F. Gazdar)	27, 31	No
NCI-H358	National Cancer Institute (A.F. Gazdar)	27,28,31	No
<u>Large Cell Carcinoma</u>			
NCI-H460	National Cancer Institute (A.F. Gazdar)	27,28	Unknown

(Continued)

TABLE 1 (Continued)

Histology Cell Line	Institution (Source*)	Reference	Prior Chemotherapy**
SMALL CELL LUNG CANCER (SCLC)			
"Classic" SCLC			
NCI-H69	National Cancer Institute (A.F. Gazdar)	26,28	Yes
NCI-H146	National Cancer Institute (A.F. Gazdar)	26,28	Yes
"Variant" SCLC			
NCI-H82	National Cancer Institute (A.F. Gazdar)	28	Yes
NCI-H524	National Cancer Institute (A.F. Gazdar)	28	Yes
"Adherent" SCLC			
DMS 114	Dartmouth Medical School (O.S. Pettengill)	32,33	No
COLON CANCER			
DLD-1	Brown University (ATCC)	34	Unknown
HCC 2998	M.D. Anderson Hospital & Tumor Institute (I.J. Fidler)	–	Unknown
HT-29	Memorial Sloan-Kettering Cancer Center (NCI-TB)	30	Unknown
LoVo	M.D. Anderson Hopsital & Tumor Institute (ATCC)	35	Unknown
SW 620	Scott White Clinic (ATCC)	36	Unknown
RENAL CANCER			
A498	National Cancer Institute (ATCC)	25	Unknown
A704	National Cancer Institute (ATCC)	25	Unknown
Caki-1	Memorial Sloan-Kettering Cancer Center (MSK)	30	Unknown

TABLE 1 (Continued)

Histology Cell Line	Institution (Source*)	Reference	Prior Chemotherapy**
SN12 K1	M.D. Anderson Hospital & Tumor Institute (I.J. Fidler)	37	Unknown
UO-31	National Cancer Institute (W.M. Linehan)	–	No

MELANOMA

LOX	Norsk Hydro's Institute Norway (O. Fodstad)	38	Unknown
Malme-3M	Memorial Sloan-Kettering Cancer Center (ATCC)	30	Unknown
RPMI-7951	Roswell Park Memorial Institute (ATCC)	39	Unknown
SK-MEL-2	Memorial Sloan-Kettering Cancer Center (ATCC)	30	Unknown
SK-MEL-5	Memorial Sloan-Kettering Cancer Center (ATCC)	40	Unknown

OVARIAN CANCER

A2780	National Cancer Institute (T.C. Hamilton)	41	No
OVCAR-3	National Cancer Institute (T.C. Hamilton)	41,42	Yes
OVCAR-4	National Cancer Institute (T.C. Hamilton)	41,42	Yes
OVCAR-5	National Cancer Institute (T.C. Hamilton)	41,42	No
OVCAR-8	National Cancer Institute (T.C. Hamilton)	–	Yes

LEUKEMIA

CCRF-CEM	Children's Cancer Research Foundation (ATCC)	43,44	Yes
HL-60	National Cancer Institute (ATCC)	45	Unknown

(Continued)

TABLE 1 (Continued)

Histology Cell Line	Institution (Source*)	Reference	Prior Chemotherapy**
K-562	University of Tennessee (ATCC)	46	Unknown
Molt-4	Roswell Park Memorial Inst. (ATCC)	47	Yes
CNS CANCER			
SNB19	Nat. Inst. Neur. & Comm. Dis. & Stroke (P.L. Kornblith)	48,49	Unknown
SNB44	Nat. Inst. Neur. & Comm. Dis. & Stroke (P.L. Kornblith)	48,49	Unknown
SNB75	Nat. Inst. Neur. & Comm. Dis. & Stroke (P.L. Kornblith)	–	Unknown
TE671	Children's Hospital, Los Angeles (NCI-TB)	50	No
U251	University of Uppsala, Sweden (NCI-TB)	51	Unknown
Miscellaneous			
MCF-7	Michigan Cancer Foundation (K. Cowan)	52	No
MCF-7/ADR	National Cancer Institute (K. Cowan)	53	Yes
P388	National Cancer Institute (NCI-TB)	54	No
P388/ADR	Southern Research Institute (NCI-TB)	54	Yes

*Cell line sources if other than original investigator were as follows: (ATCC) = American Type Culture Collection; (MSK) = Memorial Sloan-Kettering Cancer Center (Walker Laboratory); and (NCI-TB) = NCI-Division of Cancer Treatment Tumor Bank

**Prior chemotherapy status was determined from published descriptions of the cell lines or by correspondence with original investigators.

CONCLUSIONS

The available data support the appropriateness of the methods developed for in vitro drug screening and the feasibility of large scale antitumor drug screening using disease-oriented panels of human tumor cell lines. Feasibility has been demonstrated by the reproducibility of assay results and the capacity of the test system as established in a pilot-scale screening mode.

It should be recognized that the central goal of the in vitro based, disease-oriented screening program is to identify new antitumor drug candidates which would not have been discovered by the previous screening programs. Clinical testing of such new leads will ultimately provide the only means to establish or disprove the validity of the new-screen for identifying new drugs active against the common refractory human solid tumors. The ability of the screen to predict tumor-type selective activity preclinically and which may be reflected in similar selectivity in the clinic will also be an issue of major interest for retrospective analysis.

ACKNOWLEDGEMENTS

We thank the following individuals for providing samples of the cell lines described in this report: Dr. Isiah Fidler (HT-29, A549, HCC 2998 and SN12 K1), Dr. Oystein Fodstad (EKVX and LOX), Dr. Kenneth Cowan (MCF-7 and MCF-7/Adriamycin Resistant), Dr. Paul Kornblith (SNB19, SNB44, and SNB75), Dr. Marston Linnehan (UO-31), Drs. John Minna, Adi Gazdar, and Herbert Oie (lung cancer cell lines designated NCI-H...), Drs. Robert Ozols and Thomas Hamilton (OVCAR lines), and Dr. Olive Pettengill (DMS 114). Samples of other cell lines were obtained from the American Type Culture Collection, Rockville, MD, USA. We also acknowledge the expert assistance of the technical staff of the in vitro screening project at NCI-FCRF and the assistance of Mrs. Kathy Gill in preparation of this manuscript.

REFERENCES

1. Hamburger AW. Use of in vitro tests in predictive cancer chemotherapy. JNCI 66:981-988, 1981.

2. Selby P, Buick RN, and Tannock I. A critical appraisal of the "human tumor stem cell assay". N Engl J Med 308:129-134, 1983.

3. Von Hoff DD, Clark GM, Stodgill BJ, et al. Prospective clinical trial of a human tumor cloning system. Cancer Res 43:1926-1931, 1983.

4. Shoemaker RH, Wolpert-DeFilippes MK, and Venditti JM. Potentials and drawbacks of the human tumor stem cell assay. Behring Inst Mitt 74:262-272, 1984.

5. Rockwell S. Effects of clumps and clusters on survival measurements with clonogenic assays. Cancer Res 45:1601-1607, 1985.

6. Shoemaker RH, Wolpert-DeFilippes MK, Kern DH, et al. Application of a human tumor colony-forming assay to new drug screening. Cancer Res 45:2145-2153, 1985.

7. Makuch RW. Interpreting clonogenic assay results. Lancet 2:438, 1982.

8. Rozencweig M, Staquet M. Predictive tests for the response to cancer chemotherapy: Limitations related to the prediction of rare events. Cancer Treat Rep 68:611-612, 1984.

9. Salmon SE, Hamburger AW, Soehnlen B, et al. Quantitation of differential sensitivity of human-tumor stem cells to anticancer drugs. N Engl J Med 298:1321-1327, 1978.

10. Von Hoff DD, Casper J, Bradley E, et al. Association between human tumor colony forming assay results and response of an individual patient's tumor to chemotherapy. Am J Med 70:1027-1032, 1981.

11. Moon TE, Salmon SE, White CS, et al. Quantitative association between the in vitro human tumor stem cell assay and clinical response to therapy. Cancer Chemother Pharmacol 6:211-218, 1981.

12. Tveit KM, Fodstad O, Lutsberg J, et al. Colony growth and chemosensitivity in vitro of human melanoma biopsies: Relationship to clinical parameters. Int J. Cancer 29:533-538, 1982.

13. Bertelsen CA, Sondak VK, Mann BD, et al. Chemosensitivity testing of human solid tumors a review of 1582 assays with 258 clinical correlations. Cancer 53:12140-1245, 1984.

14. Meyskens FL Jr., Loescher L., Moon TE, et al. Relation of in vitro colony survival to clinical response in a prospective trial of single-agent chemotherapy for metastatic melanoma. J. Clin Oncol 2:1223-1228, 1984.

15. Sondak VK, Bertelson CA, Tanigawa N, et al. Clinical correlations with chemosensititives measured in a rapid thymidine incorporation assay. Cancer Res. 44: 1725-1728, 1984.

16. Shimizu E. Saijo N, Kanzawa F, et al. Correlation between drug sensitivity determined by clonogenic cell assay and clinical effect of chemotherapy in patients with primary lung cancer. Gann 75:1030-1035, 1984.

17. Dettrich CH, Jakes ZR, Wrba F, et al. The human tumour cloning assay in the management of breast cancer patients. Br J Cancer 52:197-203, 1985.

18. Jones SE, Dean JC, Young LA, et al. The human tumor clonogenic assay in human breast cancer. J. Clin Oncol 3:92-97, 1985.

19. Bosanquet AG, Bird MC, Price WJP, et al. An assessment of short-term tumour chemosensitivity assay in chronic lymphocytic leukemia. Br J Cancer 47:781-789, 1983.

20. Bird MC Bosanquet AG, and Gilby ED. In vitro determination of tumour chemosensitivity in haematological malignancies. Hematol Oncol 3:1-9, 1985.

21. Weisenthal LM, Dill PL, Finklestein JZ, et al. Laboratory detection of primary and acquired drug resistance in human lymphatic neoplasms. Cancer Treat Rep 70:1283-95, 1986.

22. Boyd M, Shoemaker R, Alley M, et al. New NCI disease-oriented drug screening program. Proc. Fifth NCI-EORTC Symposium on New Drugs in Cancer Therapy, Amsterdam, The Netherlands, 1986.

23. Boyd MR, Shoemaker RH, McLemore TL, Johnston MR, Alley MC, Scudiero DA, Monks A, Fine DL, Mayo JG, and Chabner BA. New Drug Development. IN: J.A. Roth, J.C. Ruckdescel and T.H. Weisenburger (eds), Thoracic Oncology, Chap. 51. New York: W.B. Saunders Co., (In press, 1987).

24. Shoemaker RH, McLemore TL, Abbott BJ, et al. Human tumor xenograft models for use with an in-vitro based, disease-oriented antitumor drug screening program. In: Human Tumor Xenografts in Anticancer Drug Development H M Pinedo, MJ Peckham, and B. Winograd (Eds) European School of Oncology Milan, (In press, 1987).

25. Giard DJ, Aaronson SA, Todaro GJ, Arnstein P, Kersey JH, Dosik H, and Parks WP. In vitro cultivation of human tumors: Establishment of cell lines derived from a series of solid tumors. J. Nat. Cancer Inst. 51:1417-1423, 1973.

26. Gazdar, AF, Carney DN, Russell EK, Sims HL, Baylin, SB, Bunn, Jr. PA, Guccion JG, and Minna JD. Establishment of continuous, clonable cultures of small-cell carcinoma of the lung which have amine precurson uptake and decarboxylation cell properties. Cancer Reearch 40:3502-3507, 1980

27. Carney DN, Gazdar AF, Bepler G, Guccion JG, Marangos PJ, Moody TW, Zweig MH, and Minna JD. Establishment and identification of small cell lung cancer cell lines having classic and variant features. Cancer Research 45:2913-2923, 1985.

28. Brower M, Carney DN, Oie HK, Gazdar AF, and Minna JD. Growth of cell lines and clinical specimens of human non-small cell lung cancer in a serum-free defined medium. Cancer Research 46:798-806, 1986.

29. Gazdar AF, and Oie HK. Cell culture methods for human lung cancer. Cancer Genetics and Cytogenetics 19:5-10, 1986.

30. Fogh J, and Trempe G. "New human tumor cell lines", Chap. 5 IN: J. Fogh (ed.) Human Tumor Cells In Vitro, pp. 115-159. New York: Plenum Publishing Corp., 1975.

31. Falzon M, McMahon JB, Gazdar AF, and Schuller HM. Pre ferential metabolism of N-nitrosodiethylamine by two cell lines derived from human pulmonary adenocarcinomas. Carcinogenesis 7:17-22, 1986.

32. Pettengill OS, Sorenson GD, Wurster-Hill DH, Curphey TJ, Noll WW, Cate CC, and Maurer LH. Isolation and growth characteristics of continuous cell lines from small-cell carcinoma of the lung. Cancer 45:906-918, 1980.

33. Wurster-Hill DH, Cannizzaro LA, Pettengill OS, Sorenson GD, Cate CC and Maurer LH. Cytogenetics of small cell carcinoma of the lung. Cancer Genetics and Cytogenetics 13: 303-330, 1984.

34. Dexter DL, Barbosa JA, and Calabresi P. N, N-dimethyl-formamide-induced alteration of cell culture character-istics and loss of tumorigenicity in cultured human colon carcinoma cells. Cancer Research 39:1020-1025, 1979.

35. Drewinko B, Romsdahl MM, Yang LY, Ahern MJ and Trujillo JM. Establishment of a human carcinoembryonic antigen-producing colon adenocarcinoma cell line. Cancer Research 36:467-475, 1976.

36. Leibovitz A, Stinson JC, McCombs WB, McCoy CE, Mazur KC, and Mabry ND. Classification of human colorectal adeno-carcinoma cell lines. Cancer Research 36:4562-45-69, 1976.

37. Naito S, von Eschenbach AC, Giazvazzi R, and Fidler, IJ. Growth and metastasis of tumor cells isolated from a human renal cell carcinoma implanted into different organs of nude mice. Complete reference.

38. Fodstad O, Aamdal S, Tveit KM, and Pihl A. Lung colony formation in adult nude mice upon intravenous injection of cells from a human melanoma xenograft. Proc Amer Assoc Cancer Res (23):881, 1982.

39. Hay RJ, Macy M, Corman-Weinblatt A, Chen TR, and McClintock FM, (eds) American Type Culture Collection Catalogue of Cell Lines and Hybridomas. 5th Edition, 1985.

40. Carey TE, Takahashi T, Resnick LA, Oettgen HF, and Old LJ. Cell surface antigens of human malignant melanoma: Mixed hemadsorption assays for humoral immunity to cultured autologous melanoma cells. Proc. Natl. Acad. Sci. USA 73:3278-3282, 1976.

41. Hamilton TC, Young RC and Ozols RF. Experimental model systems of ovarian cancer: Applications to the design and evaluation of new treatment approaches. Seminars in Oncology 11:285-298, 1984.

42. Ozols RF. Phamacologic reversal of drug resistance in ovarian cancer. Seminars in Oncology 12 (Suppl. 4): 7-11, 1985.

43. Foley GE, Lazarus H, Farber S, Uzman BG, Boone BA and McCarthy RE. Continuous culture of human lymphoblasts from peripheral blood of a child with acute leukemia. Cancer 18:522-529, 1965.

44. Foley GE, Lazarus H, Farber S, Uzman BG and Adams RA. "Studies on human leukemic cells in vitro". IN: The Proliferation and Spread of Neoplastic Cells, pp. 65-97. Baltimore: Williams and Wilkins Company, 1968.

45. Collins SJ, Gallo RC, Gallagher RE. Continuous growth and differentiation of human myeloid leukemic cells in suspension culture. Nature 270:347-349, 1977.

46. Lozzio CB and Lozzio BB. Human chronic myelogenous leukemia cell-line with positive Philadelphia chromosome. Blood 45:321-334, 1975.

47. Minowada J, Ohnuma T, and Moore GE. Brief communication: Rosette-forming human lymphoid cells. I. Establishment and evidence for origin of thymus-derived lymphocytes. J Natl Cancer Inst 49:891-895, 1972.

48. Kornblith PL, and Szypko PE. Variations in response of human brain tumors to BCNU in vitro. J. Neurosurg. 48: 580-586, 1978.

49. Kornblith PL, Smith BH and Leonard LA. Response of cultured human brain tumors to nitrosoureas: Correlation with clinical data. Cancer 47:255-265, 1981.

50. McAllister RM, Isaacs H, Rongey R, Peer M, Au W, Soukup SW, and Gardner MB. Establishment of a human medullo-blastoma cell line. Int. J. Cancer 20:206-121, 1977.

51. Ponten J. "Neoplastic human glia cells in culture". Chap. 7 IN: J. Fogh (ed.) Human Tumor Cells In Vitro, pp. 175-204. New York:Plenum Publishing Corp., 1975.

52. Soule HD, Vazquez J, Long A, Albert S, and Brennan M. A human cell line from a pleural effusion derived from a breast carcinoma. J. Natl. Cancer Inst. 51:1408-1416, 1973.

53. Foster EJ, Hill JE, Keizer HJ, et al. Cross resistance (X-RES) to adriamycin (ADR) in variant cell lines of MCF-7 breast cancer selected for primary resistance to either methotrexate (MTX) or tamoxifen (TAM). Proc Am Assoc Cancer Res 23:776, 1982

54. Schabel FM Jr., Skipper HE, Trader MW, Laster Jr. WR, Griswold Jr. DP, and Corbett TH. Establishment of cross-resistance profiles for new agents. Cancer Treat. Rep. 67:905-922, 1983.

55. McLemore TL, Blacker PC, Gregg M. A novel intrapulmonary model for the orthotopic propagation of human lung cancers in athymic nude mice. Cancer Res (In press, 1987).

56. Shoemaker R, Wolpert-DeFilippes M, Mayo J., et. al. Experimental chemotherapy studies of a human melanoma in nude mice using a survival endpoint. Proc. Amer. Assoc. Cancer Res 26:330, 1985.

57. Houchens, DP, Ovejera AA, Riblet SM, and Slagel DE. Human brain tumor xenografts in nude mice as a chemotherapy model. Eur J Cancer Clin Oncol 19:799-805, 1983.

58. Chabner BA, Clendeninn NJ, Curt GA. Symposium on cellular resistance to anticancer drugs. Introduction. Cancer Treat Rep 67:855-7, 1983.

59. Straus FH, Chernois ND, and Straus E. Demonstration of reducing enzyme systems in neoplasms and living mammalian tissues by triphenyl-tetrazolium chloride. Science 108: 113-115, 1948.

60. Nineham AW. The chemistry of formazans and tetrazolium salts. Chemistry Reviews 55:355-483, 1955.

61. Pearse AGE. Principles of oxidoreductase histochemistry, Chap. 20, IN: Histochemistry, Theoretical and Applies, 3rd Edition, Churchill Livingston, Edinburgh, 1972.

62. Black MM, and Speer FD. Further observations on the effects of cancer chemotherapeutic agents on the in vitro dehydrogenase activity of cancer tissue. J. Natl. Cancer Inst. 14:1147-1158, 1954.

63. Mosmann T. Rapid colorimetric assay for cellular growth and survival: Application to proliferation and cytotoxicity assays. J Immunol. Meth. 65:55-63, 1983.

64. Alley MC, Scudiero DA, Monks A, Czerwinski MJ, Shoemaker RH, and Boyd MR. Validation of an automated microculture tetrazolium assay (MTA) to assess growth and drug sensitivity of human tumor cell lines. Proc. Am Assoc Cancer Res 27:389, 1986.

65. Cole, S.P.C. Rapid chemosensitivity testing of human lung tumor cell lines. Cancer Chemother Pharmacol 17:259-263, 1986.

66. Carmichael J, DeGraff WG, Gazdar AF, Minna JD, and Mitchell JB. Evaluation of a tetrazolium-based semiautomated colormetric assay: assessment of chemosensitivity testing. Cancer Research 47: 936-942, 1987.

67. Scudiero D, Shoemaker R, Paull K, et al. A new tetrazolium reagent for a simplified growth and drug sensitivity assay of human tumor cell lines. Proc Am Assoc Cancer Res 28:421, 1987.

Prediction of Response to Cancer Therapy, pages 287-293
© 1988 Alan R. Liss, Inc.

CELLULAR GLUTATHIONE LEVELS AND SENSITIVITY TO RADIATION AND ANTINEOPLASTIC AGENTS IN HUMAN OVARIAN CANCER

Robert F. Ozols, Thomas C. Hamilton and Robert C. Young
Experimental Therapeutics Section, Medicine Branch, National Cancer Institute, Bethesda, Maryland 20892 U.S.A.

INTRODUCTION

Glutathione (GSH) is a tripeptide thiol found in virtually all mammalian cells. The role of GSH metabolism in the determination of antineoplastic drug cytotoxicity and radiation sensitivity has been recently reviewed (Meister, 1983: Arrick, 1984). GSH is involved in a number of biochemical pathways which may alter the cytotoxicity of both radiation and antineoplastic drugs. However, the precise mechanism by which GSH modulates the cytotoxicity of some antineoplastic agents and of radiation remains to be established and indeed it is not certain that the same mechanism is responsible for mediating the effects of different agents. Among the mechanisms which have been studied are the reaction of GSH with cytotoxic electrophiles leading to inactive conjugates, the elimination of hydrogen peroxide and free radicals generated by antineoplastic drugs and radiation and the repair of lethal damage done to biologically important molecules (primarily DNA) by antineoplastic drugs and radiation. Studies on the metabolism of GSH and its correlation with antineoplastic drug and radiation cytotoxicity have been stimulated by the recent observation that there exists potentially clinically useful ways to manipulate GSH levels.

On the basis of initial reports (Relle-Somfai, 1984) that melphalan resistant L1210 cells had 2 to 4-fold higher GSH levels than sensitive cells and that reduction of GSH levels led to restoration of melphalan sensitivity, we have studied the role of GSH metabolism in human ovarian cancer cell lines with particular emphasis on the modification of radiation survival parameters and cisplatin and melphalan cytotoxicity.

MATERIALS AND METHODS

We have established a series of human ovarian cancer cell lines from previously untreated patients and from patients clinically resistant to chemotherapy (Hamilton, 1984). In addition, we have developed a series of cell lines with primary resistance to melphalan (Green, 1984), cisplatin (Behrens, 1987) and adriamycin (Rogan, 1984) by stepwise incubation of A2780 (the sensitive cell line derived from an untreated patient) with melphalan, cisplatin, and adriamycin. These sublines are approximately 7-10 fold, 10-70 fold, and 10-150 fold more resistant to the respective drugs than the parent line (A2780).

In addition, we have adapted one of the cell lines (OVCAR-3) established from a drug resistant patient (Hamilton, 1983) for intraperitoneal growth in nude mice (Hamilton, 1985). In this in vivo model system, the mice die of disseminated ovarian cancer with intraabdominal carcinomatosis and ascites. These in vitro and in vivo model system have allowed us to study the selective cytotoxicity and potential therapeutic advantage of agents which can modify antineoplastic drug activity.

Buthionine sulfoximine (BSO), a specific inhibitor of GSH synthesis (Griffith, 1979), was evaluated in vitro and in vivo as a potentiator of alkylating agent and cisplatin cytotoxicity. In addition, BSO was used to study radiation survival parameters in the antineoplastic drug sensitive and resistant cell lines, Table 1.

RESULTS

In Vitro Modification of Drug Cytotoxicity by BSO

Table 2 summarizes the effects of BSO upon melphalan and cisplatin cytotoxicity in cell lines with acquired resistance in vitro to melphalan and cisplatin as well as in the cell line OVCAR-3 established from a patient who re-

ceived prior therapy with cisplatin, adriamycin and cytoxan. All the drug resistant cell lines studied had higher
levels of GSH compared to the sensitive cell lines. In
addition, both in cell lines with acquired resistance in
vitro to cisplatin and to melphalan as well as in the cell
line established from a patient who was clinically resistant to these agents, BSO produced a dose modifying effect
upon melphalan and cisplatin cytotoxicity.

TABLE 1. Ovarian Carcinoma Cell Lines

From Untreated Patients

A1847*
A2780*
NIH:OVCAR-5

From Refractory Patients

Cell Line	Drugs
NIH:OVCAR-2	Cyclophosphamide, cisplatin, hemamethyl-melamine, irradiation
NIH-OVCAR-3	Cyclophosphamide, cisplatin, adriamycin
NIH-OVCAR-4	Cyclophosphamide, cisplatin, adriamycin

Resistance Induced In Vitro

Drug Resistant Variant Cell Line

(Ratio of IC_{50} of resistant line to IC_{50} for sensitive parent line)

Parent Cell Line	Melphalan	Adriamycin	Cisplatin
A1847	1847ME	1847AD	1847CP
	(4)	(5)	(3)
A2780	2780ME	2780AD	2780CP
	(10)	(150)	(10-70)

---

*Kindly provided by Dr. Stuart Aaronson, NCI

Table 2. Effect of BSO Upon Cytotoxicity In Vitro

Cell Line	GSH Level (nmol/10^6 cells)	Dose Modification Melphalan	Cisplatin
2780ME	4.8	3.4	1.8
2780^{CP}	6.1	6.3	3.2
OVCAR-3	15.1	3.2	2.0

From Hamilton, 1985 and Ozols, 1987.

Effect of BSO In Vivo Upon Melphalan Cytotoxicity

We first examined the effect of oral BSO on mouse tissue GSH content and OVCAR-3 ascites GSH content in the nude mouse model system of ovarian cancer previously described, Table 3 (Ozols, 1987). Note that BSO produced a decrease in GSH levels to essentially the same degree in bone marrow, gastrointestinal mucosa, and ascites cells.

TABLE 3. Effect of Oral L-BSO on Mouse Tissue GSH Content and OVCAR-3 Ascites GSH Content

Tissue	Control GSH Content Mean ($\pm$ 1SD)	GSH Content After Oral L-BSO Mean ($\pm$ 1SD)	Percent Reduction
Bone Marrow	0.33 $\pm$ 0.10	0.07 $\pm$ 0.02	79
Gastro-intestinal Mucosa (nmol/mg DNA)	0.52 $\pm$ 0.11	0.06 $\pm$ 0.02	88
Ascites (nmol/10^6 cells)	12.36 $\pm$ 1.51	0.54 $\pm$ 0.22	96

Nude mice were inoculated with 40 x 10^6 OVCAR-3 ovarian cancer cells and after 2 days placed on drinking water that contained 30 mM L-BSO. Five days later GSH levels were measured in tumor cells and in normal tissues. [From Ozols et al. (1987).

However, BSO did not potentiate the LD_{10} dose of melphalan in normal non-tumor bearing nude mice. BSO, however, did potentiate the cytotoxicity in vivo of melphalan in this nude mouse model. Melphalan was administered at a time when tumors were well established in the host (8 days after inoculation of 40×10^6 tumor cells I.P.). In this model of human ovarian carcinoma, there is a dose dependent effect of melphalan on survival. The median survival times (MST) with 5 and 10 mg/kg doses were 75 and 102.5 days. The MST for control animals was 46 days. Administration of BSO orally in the drinking water for 5 days had no effect on survival. BSO treatment of tumor bearing mice prior to the administration of melphalan (5 mg/kg) increased the MST to 205 days. In addition, there were 3/15 long-term survivors in mice treated with 10 mg/kg melphalan plus BSO, whereas there was only 1 long term survivor in the group treated with melphalan alone (Ozols, 1987).

Modification of Radiation Survival Parameters by BSO

The D_0 for A2780 was 101 with an n of 1.40 as determined from radiation survival curves using clonogenicity in soft agar (Louie, 1985). In contrast, 2780ME has a D_0 of 146 and an n of 2.12 while 2780^{CP} has a D_0 of 187 and an n of 1.62. It is of particular note that there was no statistically significant difference in radiation survival parameters for the 2780^{AD} resistant cell line. Depletion of intracellular GSH by a 48 hour monolayer exposure to BSO followed by maintenance of the GSH depleted state by the presence of BSO in the cloning media led to a marked sensitization of 2780ME. The D_0 decreased from 143 to 95. Similarly for the cisplatin resistant cell line BSO also produced sensitization to radiation with the D_0 changing from 183 to 134.

DISCUSSION

These results demonstrate that cellular GSH levels are an important determinant of the responsiveness of human ovarian cancer cells to radiation and to cisplatin and melphalan. Patients with ovarian cancer who become resistant to therapy develop broad cross-resistance between alkylating agents, cisplatin and irradiation. The observation that in a clinically relevant experimental model system of human ovarian cancer, BSO can potentiate the cytotoxic effects of melphalan leading to a marked prolongation in survival has led to the preclinical evaluation of BSO and toxicology studies prior to clinical trials in drug resistant patients.

Since BSO decreases GSH levels in normal tissues as well as in tumor cells, it is apparent that clinical trials with BSO must be conducted in a careful manner in an effort not to exacerbate the toxic effects of the antineoplastic agents. Specifically, it has been demonstrated in our nude mouse system that BSO potentiates the toxicity of cisplatin and consequently, this combination may not be clinically useful in patients with ovarian cancer. However, it is possible that cisplatin and BSO could be administered intraperitoneally and then systemic toxicity could be decreased or eliminated by the intravenous infusion of glutathione ester. These studies are being modeled in the experimental systems of ovarian cancer. In addition, we could not demonstrate any enhancement of the toxicity of carboplatin in the nude mouse model system of ovarian cancer. BSO also potentiates the cytotoxicity of carboplatin in a similar manner as it does cisplatin in vitro in human ovarian cancer cell lines. Consequently, BSO plus carboplatin may be a potentially useful combination in ovarian cancer patients.

The exact mechanism responsible for the broad cross-resistance between melphalan and radiation and cisplatin remains to be established. It is possible that the common pathway relates to enhanced DNA repair capacity. We have demonstrated in the cisplatin and melphalan resistant cell lines that there is increased DNA repair (Behrens, 1987). However, the role GSH has in the repair process remains to be established.

In conclusion, cellular GSH levels are an important determinant in melphalan, cisplatin, and radiation toxicity in human ovarian cancer cells. The demonstration that BSO can selectively potentiate the cytotoxic effects of melphalan suggests that pharmacologic manipulation of BSO levels leading to an enhanced therapeutic index may be a clinical possibility in the treatment of drug resistant and radiation resistant ovarian cancer patients.

REFERENCES

Arrick BA, Nathan CF (1984). Glutathione metabolism as a determinant of therapeutic efficacy: A review. Cancer

Res 44:4224-4232.

Behrens BC, Hamilton TC, Masuda H, Grotzinger KR, Whang-Peng J, Louie KG, Knutsen T, McKoy, WM, Young RC, Ozols RF (1987). Characterization of a cisdiamminedichloroplatinum resistant human ovarian cancer cell line and its use in evaluation of platinum analogues. Cancer Res 47:414-418.

Green JA, Vistica DT, Young RC, Hamilton TC, Rogan AM, Ozols RF (1984). Potentiation of melphalan cytotoxicity in human ovarian cancer cell lines by glutathione depletion. Cancer Res 44:5427-5431.

Griffith OW, Meister A (1979). Potent and specific inhibitor of glutathione synthesis by buthionine sulfoximine (S-n-butyl homocysteine sulfoximine). J Biol Chem 253: 7558-7560.

Hamilton TC, Young RC, McKoy WM, Grotzinger KR, Green JA, Chu EW, Whang-Peng J, Rogan AM, Green WA, Ozols RF (1983). Characterization of a human ovarian carcinoma cell line (NIH: OVCAR-3) with androgen and estrogen receptors. Cancer Res 43: 5379-5389.

Hamilton TC, Young RC, Ozols RF (1984). Experimental model systems of ovarian cancer. Semin Oncol 11:285-298.

Hamilton TC, Young RC, Louie KG, Behrens BC, McKoy WM, Grotzinger KR, Ozols RF (1985). Characterization of a xenograft model of human ovarian cancer which produces ascites and intraabdominal carcinomatosis. Cancer Res 44:5286-5290.

Hamilton TC, Winker MA, Louie KG, Batist G, Behrens BC, Tsuruo T, Grotzinger KR, McKoy WM, Young RC, Ozols RF (1985). Augmentation of adriamycin, melphalan and cisplatin cytotoxicity in drug resistant and sensitive human ovarian cancer cell lines by buthionine sulfoximine mediated glutathione depletion. Biochem Pharmacol 34:2583-2586.

Louie KG, Behrens BC, Kinsella JJ, Hamilton TC, Grotzinger KR, McKoy WM, Winker MA, Ozols RF (1985). Radiation survival parameters of antineoplastic drug-sensitive and resistant human ovarian cancer cell lines and their modification by buthionine sulfoximine. Cancer Res 45:2110-2115.

Meister A (1983). Selective modification of glutathione metabolism. Science 220:472-477.

Ozols RF, Louie KG, Plowman J, Behrens BC, Fine RL, Dykes D, Hamilton TC (1987). Biochem Pharmacol 36:147-153.

Rogan AM, Hamilton TC, Young RC, Klecker R, Ozols RF (1984). Reversal of adriamycin resistance by verapamil in human ovarian cancer. Science 224:994-996.

Prediction of Response to Cancer Therapy, pages 295–298
© 1988 Alan R. Liss, Inc.

FUNDAMENTAL PROBLEMS AND FUTURE POSSIBILITIES FOR
TREATMENT PREDICTOR SYSTEMS

THOMAS C. HALL, M.D.

The University of Hawaii Cancer Center and
The Center for Molecular Medicine and
Immunology, Newark, NJ   07103

CONCLUSION

The symposium material has described the techniques,
applications and results of tests based upon varying
combination of drugs, host tumors and technical factors.
The fundamental differences appear between tests based
upon examination of the tumor or upon treatment of the
tumor. Basic differences are seen between a test which
will individualize more effective therapy, and a test
which will predict later clinical effectiveness of a
totally new drug. We have seen that some tests are drug
oriented, others tumor oriented, and that in-vitro tests
generally are less able than the subrenal test to mimic
the pharmacologic variables present in the clinical
situation.

Why has it been so much easier to define sensitivity
to anti-infectives? Among the many differences from
antibiotic screening include the poor in vitro growth
rates of tumors; difficulty of testing combination
therapies in vitro; absence of the pharmacologic
contribution of the host from cell culture systems;
bacterial growth fraction which aproaches 100% vs <10% for
solid tumor; lack of host immunologic cytotoxic responses
the cancer cells which survive chemotherapy. Figure 2
summarizes some of these problems.

Figure 1
Fundamental Problems with Soft Agar Assay

1. Non-representative of tumor
2. Does not contain normal control for T/C
3. Does not contain normal anabolizing/catabolizing
    organs
4. What grows may not be representative of primary tumor
5. Time to grow may be too long to be clinically useful
6. "Colonies" may be aggregates not single cell clones
7. Duration of drug exposure non-clinical in that it is
    too short
8. Concentrations of drug exposure non-clinical i.e. one
    level
9. Combination therapy hard to do: not enough tissues,
    drugs interact
10. Only a minority of tumors grow enough, mostly myeloma
    and ovary
11. Antimetabolites do not work; steroids do poorly
12. End points: (pH) (dye exclusion) may be poor growth
    indices

Figure 2
Fundamental Differences Between Cancer Prediction and
Microbial Sensitivity

1. Fractional kill T/C greater for antimicrobials
2. Immune system can "mop up" last logs of microbes
3. Microbial targets are not present in host: cell
    walls in bacteria; purines needed by trypanosomes
4. Microbial division rate and DNA synthesis faster
5. Growth fraction of microbes faster
6. In vitro microbe colonies resemble in vivo colonies;
    but in vivo tumor colonies do not reflect tumor
    heterogeneity
7. Infected animal models are close to the human; most
    animal, mouse intraperitoneal leukemic, cancer models
    are not analogous to human solid tumors.

The use of new predictive tests may be slowed down by the general disaffection with the soft agar tests, and it would be well to examine some of the problems that are presented by this type of test (fig 1).

In addition to these problems, there were others which characterize new therapeutic proposals generally. These include: 1) inadequate use of patient controls: i.e. not tested in patients known to be resistant to certain drugs; lack of inclusion of normal tissue in the assay, so that the dose levels chosen showed antitumor effects but were too high for clinical use; 2) inadequate clinical correlations i.e. poor follow-up of drug predictions; 3) lack of good clinical trials of drug regimens based upon positive test predictions for unexpected, unusual or even unpopular drugs; 4) unsuitability of the assay for studying combination therapy.

The main problem with tests based upon tissue constituents, such as receptors, is that each applies to only one drug, resulting in the need to do other-drug oriented tests on limited amounts of tissue.

All in vitro tests suffer from lack of sufficient assays of normal host tissue, which also bind, transport, anabolize, catabolize drugs. Such normal tissues suffer their own drug-induced toxicity, which determines what is tolerable clinically.

The in vivo rodent tests permit serial examination of the effects over time of single drugs, and combinations given at different concentrations, by several routes and at various time intervals. Because of the small volumes of tissue, they may permit cost-savings that are substantial, as compared to giving test doses to patients.

A library of constitutive data obtained from tumors at initial diagnosis might well be collected and stored for patients who are both at high risk for recurrence and for whose tumors there are agents whose activity might be predicted. Such constitutive studies could include multiple steroid receptors, P-180 proteins, oncogene products, cytogenetics, phosphorylation of antimetabolites, uptake of drugs, GSH levels, deamination and phosphorolysis.

Probably the ideal test would be one in which the patient could be treated with a few doses of the clinical agents being considered, and the effects on tumor and host measured non-invasively. The use of serial MRI measurements may help here by measuring phosphorylated drugs, or tumor and host tissue changes induced, for example, in DNA levels; however, the actual levels of drugs products or induced changes seem too low to be measured. The effect of treatment on serial uptake of trace-labelled drugs, or on drug deranged tumor synthesis of DNA, RNA or product e.g. (CEA) is an area which so far has been initially interesting, and later may become more relevant. The use of radionuclides in humans, or the administration of small amounts of drugs to patients prior to surgery has occasionally been reported and has great potential value. However, the matter of patient protection against drug or radionuclide late effects needs to be carefully addressed.

In summary, the apparently great potential for predictive tests has yet to be realized in cancer therapy. Presently, the primary need for a human screen for new preclinical agents seems best addressed by the new NCI screen and the new soft-agar solid matrix in vitro tests. The renal subcapsular test best serves our clinical need to select the best single agent or combination for a particular patient. The most exciting and underused existing systems involve preoperative injection of small amounts of agents and examination of drug uptake and drug-induced perturbations in synthesis of macromolecules such as DNA. The most promising systems involve non-invasive study of differentiated uptake of radiolabelled tracer doses of drugs and the observation of their effects on host tissues e.g. by MRI.

The deteriorating health care system secondary removal of federal funds from health care to the military and to the DRGs in the USA with their emphasis upon paying only for immediate care, does not presently provide funds for such tissue analyses from tumor patients. Therefore, systematic critiquing of old and new predictive tests should best be undertaken by the NCI or Cancer Centers, in order to permit ongoing systematic study of existing tests and new ones as they develop, and to facilitate their application to clinical practice.

Index